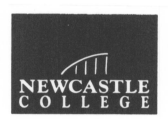

BODY TALK

BREATHING

THE RESPIRATORY SYSTEM

JENNY BRYAN

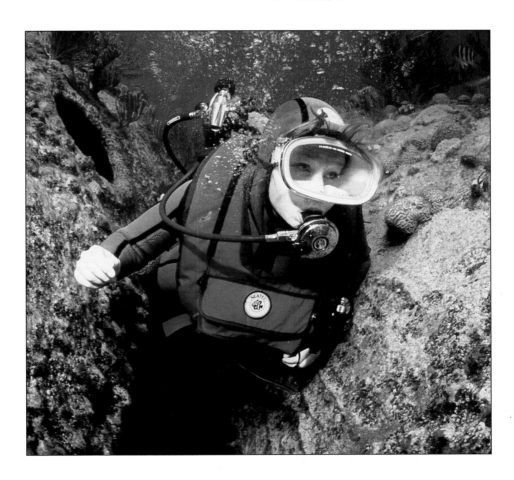

Wayland

B O D Y   T A L K

BREATHING

DIGESTION

MIND AND MATTER

MOVEMENT

REPRODUCTION

SMELL, TASTE AND TOUCH

SOUND AND VISION

THE PULSE OF LIFE

Editor: Catherine Baxter
Series Design: Loraine Hayes
Consultant: Dr Tony Smith – Associate Editor of the *British Medical Journal*
Cover and title page: Diver with oxygen tank.

First published in 1992 by Wayland (Publishers) Ltd,
61 Western Road, Hove, BN3 1JD, England.

British Library Cataloguing in Publication Data

Bryan, Jenny
Breathing. – (Body Talk Series)
I. Title II. Series
612.2

ISBN 0-7502-0490-7

Typeset by Key Origination, 1 Commercial Road, Eastbourne
Printed in Italy by G. Canale & C.S.p.A., Turin

CONTENTS

Introduction   4

The first breath   6

How air gets into the blood   8

Why we need oxygen   10

Breathing properly   12

The brain and breathing   14

The nose   17

Colds and flu   19

Smoking   22

The tobacco industry   24

Air pollution   26

Air-conditioning   28

Chest disorders   30

Asthma   32

Tuberculosis   34

Cystic fibrosis   36

Anaesthetic gases   38

Artificial ventilation   40

Better breathing   42

Does all life need oxygen?   44

Glossary   46

Books to read   47

Index   48

INTRODUCTION

WANTED: two spongy bags for gas processing. Must be highly flexible and able to work under great pressure. Very long-term contract. Should expect to be mistreated.

Not a very attractive job description is it? But those are the conditions under which our lungs must work. They must inflate and deflate about 20,000 times a day, 365 days a year so that air can enter our bodies and provide a constant supply of life-giving oxygen to our cells.

The same principles of breathing can be seen in all birds, mammals, fish and insects, though the mechanisms may vary. Oxygen is taken out of the air, taken into the bloodstream, carried to all the cells in the body and used to produce energy. Waste gas - carbon dioxide - is then carried back to the lungs and expelled into the atmosphere.

Humans breathe in through their noses and, sometimes, their mouths. The nose is better designed for the job since it warms and filters the air before it passes down into the throat (pharynx), and on through the voice box (larynx).

Below the throat, two long tubes lie alongside each other. One - the trachea - carries air to the lungs. The other - the oesophagus - carries food to the stomach. So that there is no mistake, the opening to the voice box has a cover called the epiglottis. This flips open to allow air down but slams shut to keep food out.

At its lower end, the trachea splits into two. One tube - the left bronchus - goes to the left lung, and the right bronchus takes air to the right lung. Each bronchus divides into smaller and smaller passages, called bronchioles. At the end of the smallest tubes are tiny air sacs, called alveoli, where the real business of gas processing goes on.

It is the alveoli which pay the price for our thoughtlessness. They must deal with the gases from car exhausts and factory chimneys. They are also assaulted every day by the poisonous chemicals in cigarette smoke.

No wonder those bouncy sponges that start out as efficient gas processors, often end up worn out and unable to give the body the oxygen it needs.

This is what the insides of your lungs look like. The large opening at the left of the picture is a bronchiole. The smaller, spongy sections on the right are the alveoli where gas exchange takes place. You can see how fragile the tissue is and how easily it might be damaged.

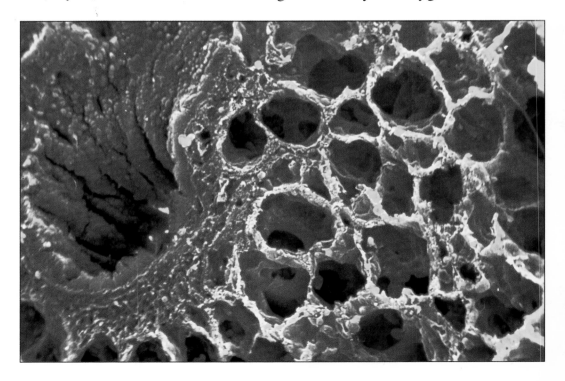

The respiratory system

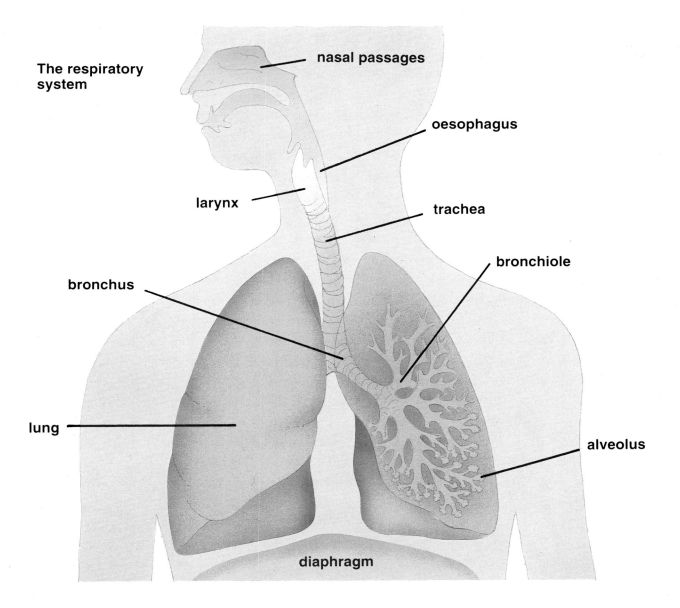

nasal passages

oesophagus

larynx

trachea

bronchiole

bronchus

lung

alveolus

diaphragm

RIGHT These are lungs from sheep. The healthy looking lungs on the left came from an Australian sheep. The diseased lungs on the right came from a Kuwaiti sheep. It died as a result of breathing in (inhaling) large amounts of crude oil from the wells left burning by retreating Iraqi soldiers at the end of the 1991 Gulf War.

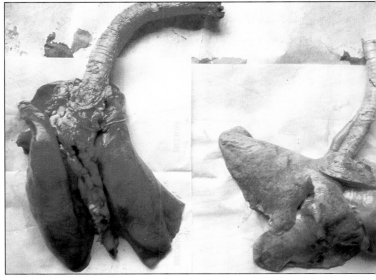

THE FIRST BREATH

Before birth a foetus relies on its mother's blood to take oxygen to its cells and carry carbon dioxide away. Its lungs are filled with fluid and don't have to breathe although they do take a few practice breaths as birth approaches.

At birth, a baby's lungs must fill with air for the first time. They can't do this on their own. Breathing is controlled by muscles that let the chest expand and the lungs inflate.

First, the baby's brain realizes that oxygen is no longer coming from the mother and it must act quickly to start the baby breathing. The brain sends messages down nerves to the intercostal muscles between the ribs and the diaphragm - a sheet of muscle that lies below the lungs and separates the chest from the stomach. Occasionally something goes wrong at this stage, so doctors keep respiratory equipment close at hand.

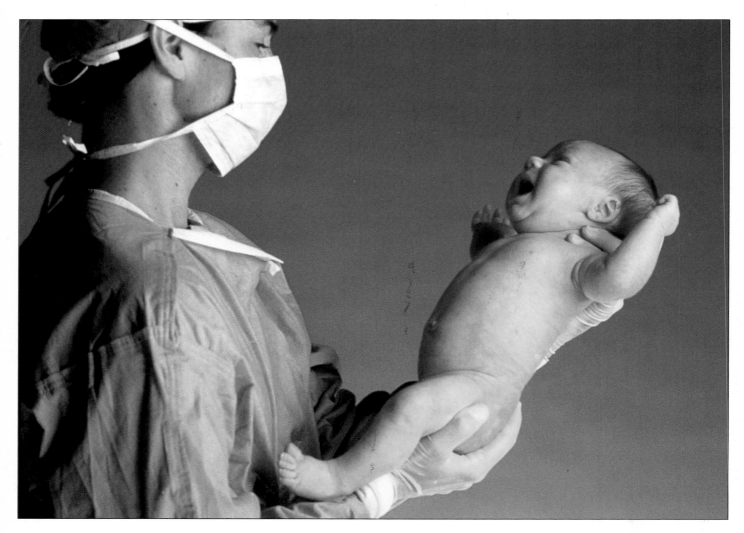

This baby's first cries have helped open up its lungs and start it breathing.

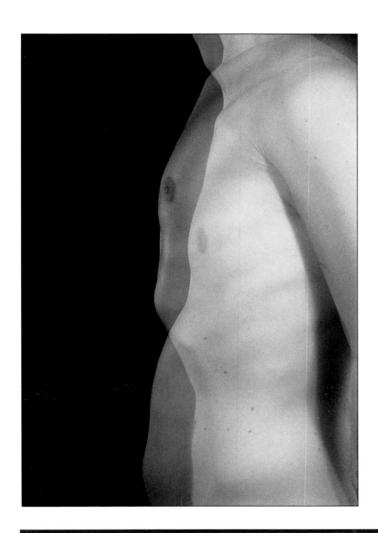

But, all being well, these messages tell the intercostal muscles to pull the rib cage outwards and the diaphragm to relax downwards so the space in the chest gets bigger. This makes the pressure in the chest go down to less than atmospheric pressure so air rushes in to fill the lungs.

To breathe out, the muscles go into reverse. The space in the chest gets smaller and the pressure rises, pushing air out of the lungs. The whole process then begins all over again.

If the insides of the lungs were dry, the effort needed to inflate them would be too much for the baby. Cells in the lungs continually make a detergent-like substance, called surfactant. This lubricates (oils) the lungs and makes it easier for the inner surfaces to slide over one another and open up to let air in.

LEFT Look how far the chest expands when you breathe in and the abdomen extends when you breathe out. All the movements depend on the muscles between the ribs and the diaphragm – which is below the rib cage.

WHEN THE LUNGS ARE TOO SMALL

One in 100 babies is born with a condition called respiratory distress syndrome. This means that their lungs have not fully developed and they cannot produce enough surfactant. The problem is most common in premature babies, especially those born ten or more weeks too early. Without enough surfactant, the premature baby is simply not strong enough to breathe. So it has to be attached to a machine, called a ventilator, which breathes for it (right).

Recently, doctors have discovered how to make surfactant. So premature babies can be given it to help them breathe. Twenty years ago, about half the babies born with respiratory distress syndrome died. But thanks to modern treatment, including surfactant therapy, 90 per cent now survive.

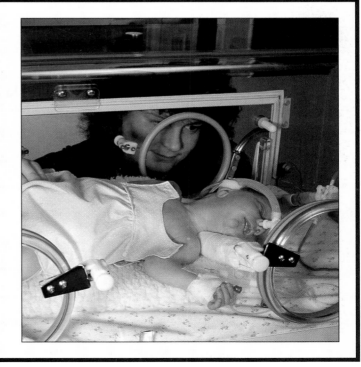

HOW AIR GETS INTO THE BLOOD

An average human lung contains about 300 million alveoli. If all the alveoli in both lungs were spread out they would cover an area of about 80 square metres. It's hard to believe, but that's about the size of a tennis court!

Criss-crossing the walls of all the tiny alveoli are even tinier hair-like blood vessels called capillaries. It is through these that oxygen is absorbed into the bloodstream and carbon dioxide passed back into the lungs. The walls of the alveoli are paper thin. This means that the molecules of oxygen and carbon dioxide have to travel less than a thousandth of a millimetre – a minute distance – to get in and out of the blood.

Oxygen and carbon dioxide do not simply float around in the blood. They are carried about by red blood cells on a chemical called haemoglobin. This is also the pigment that makes blood red.

Blood arrives in the capillaries of the alveoli from the right side of the heart. This means it has

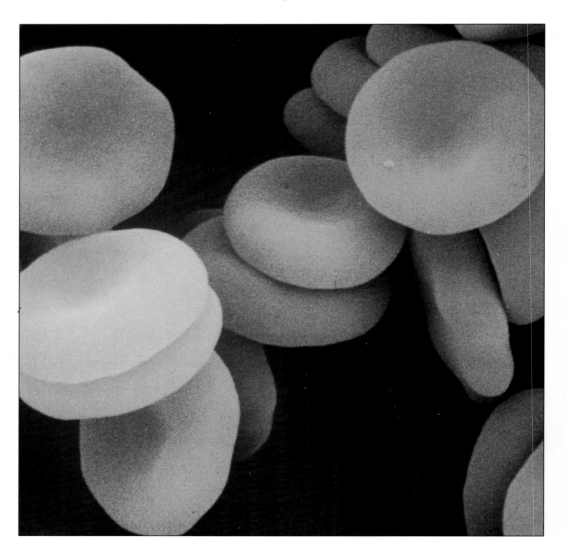

This photograph of red blood cells was taken under a microscope. A false colour was then added to make the cells show up. Mature red blood cells carry oxygen around the body. Their shape enables maximum amounts of oxygen and carbon dioxide to be exchanged.

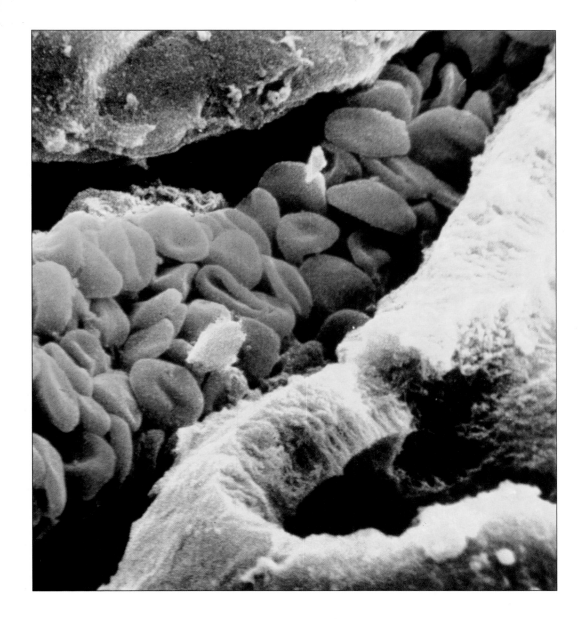

All day, every day, gas exchange goes on across the walls of the capillaries of the alveoli deep inside the lungs. As one lot of newly oxygenated blood sets off back to the heart, ready to go around the body, the next batch arrives ready to unload its carbon dioxide and take on fresh supplies of oxygen.

already been all around the body and its oxygen has been used up and converted into carbon dioxide ready to be breathed out.

The capillaries are so narrow that the red cells have to squeeze through. This means that they are pressed against the capillary walls and that oxygen and carbon dioxide swap places. Molecules of carbon dioxide come out of the red blood cells across the capillary walls and into the alveoli in exchange for oxygen molecules which go in the opposite direction.

Oxygen is then carried back to the left side of the heart ready to be pumped around the body, and carbon dioxide is breathed out.

WHAT'S IN AIR?

The air you breathe in is 79 per cent nitrogen, 21 per cent oxygen and 0.04 per cent carbon dioxide. The air you breathe out contains slightly more nitrogen, 16.4 per cent oxygen and 4 per cent carbon dioxide.

There are also small amounts of pollutants in the air that you breathe. These include nitrogen dioxide and sulphur dioxide which can be harmful, especially to people with lung problems. The exact amounts of these pollutants that are in the air depend on where you live and what the weather is like at the time.

WHY WE NEED OXYGEN

Your cells, your dog's cells, your goldfish's cells, even the cells of your stick insect need oxygen. Without oxygen in the air, life, as we know it, would come to an end.

Blood that has picked up oxygen in the lungs is pumped to all parts of the body through smaller and smaller blood vessels until it reaches more tiny capillaries. There, oxygen diffuses (spreads) out into nearby cells and carbon dioxide diffuses back into the capillaries.

All cells need oxygen to produce chemical energy. They need this energy for the millions of jobs they do every single day. You don't need to be moving about for your cells to need energy. Everything you do – breathing, eating, digesting and blinking needs energy. In fact, you even need energy to think. Not the sort of amounts that you use up in a game of hockey or tennis but energy just the same.

Without oxygen, cells soon die. A few minutes without any oxygen can cause irreparable damage to the brain and other organs. Even a small reduction in oxygen can leave you panting for breath, weak and dizzy.

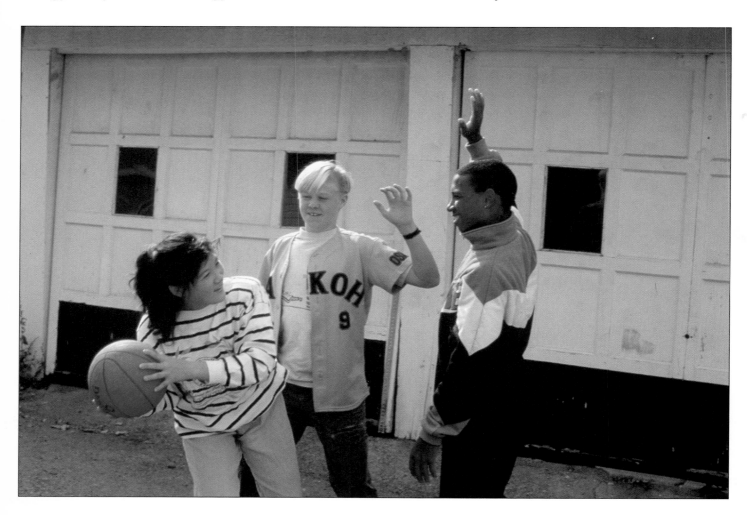

GIVING OXYGEN

In some lung diseases, the alveoli become less efficient at taking oxygen from the air. But if they are given extra oxygen they can make up the shortfall. Some people can get by with a few puffs from an oxygen cylinder every few hours. But others rely on oxygen concentrators to provide them with oxygen for several hours a day.

These machines take oxygen from the air and feed it through a long tube into the nose. They are very efficient and, with their long tubing, allow people to move about their homes freely while getting all the oxygen they need.

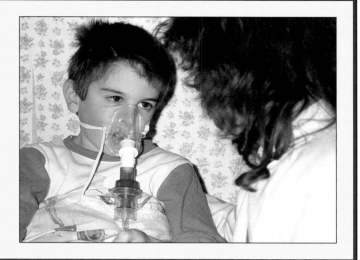

RIGHT Even when we are resting we still need oxygen.

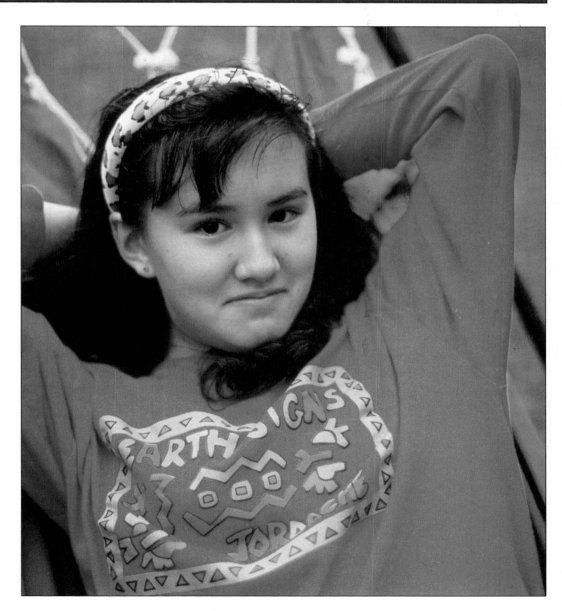

LEFT When you are exercising you breathe faster in order to get the oxygen needed to produce lots of energy.

BREATHING PROPERLY

Children breathe faster than adults. A newborn baby breathes about thirty times a minute but an adult breathes at about half that rate. When you are sitting quietly you are probably taking in about 500 ml of air in each breath - more than enough to fill a milk carton. But if you ran down the street to catch a bus you could be breathing in as much as 100 litres per minute.

Top athletes can do even better. Running flat out, some take between forty and sixty breaths a minute and breathe in over 200 litres of air during that time. They don't have bigger lungs than the rest of us. But they are much better at taking in air and getting oxygen. From 100-150 litres of air they could get around 5 litres of oxygen ready to help in energy production.

When you are breathing quietly, about two-thirds of the air you breathe in actually gets down into your lungs. The rest stays in your mouth, trachea (windpipe) and bronchi.

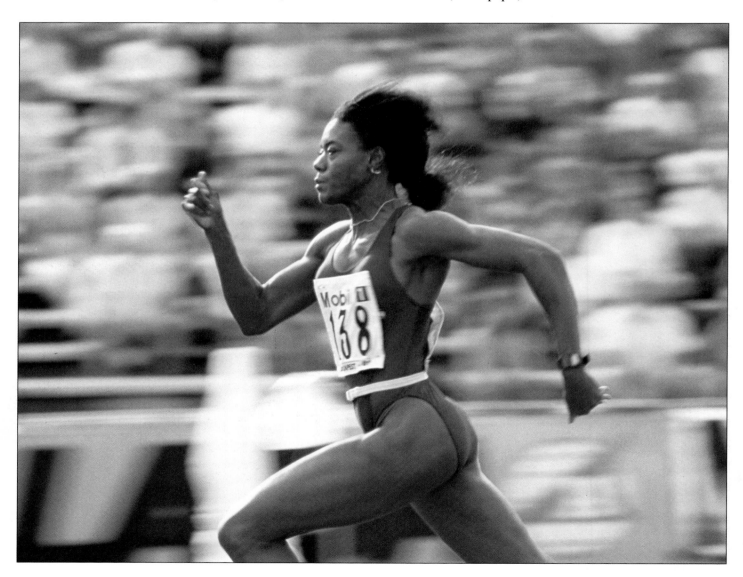

Top athletes, such as Jamaican sprinter Merlene Ottey, have to learn to breathe properly.

Your lungs always have some air in them, even between breaths. Otherwise, they would collapse. At any one time there is about 1,500 ml of air in the lungs - easily enough to fill three milk cartons. The maximum amount that you can breathe in will depend on how much you can breathe out. When learning to breathe more efficiently, athletes practise breathing out, rather than breathing in. You could bear this in mind when training for Sports Day at school.

Singers and public speakers also have to learn to breathe more efficiently. They need to be able to breathe in large amounts of air so that they don't have to take any quick breaths when they are in mid sentence. They learn to breathe from their diaphragms. They squeeze out as much air as possible and then feel their lungs fill from the bottom upwards.

People who can't get enough air into their lungs soon become breathless. Their lungs inflate and deflate more and more quickly as they try to get more air. But this leaves them with less and less time to breathe deeply. They get no more air but their breathing becomes much more of an effort. This, in turn, means that they use more energy in breathing and the shortage of oxygen gets worse. People with long-term breathing problems feel very tired and cannot move around normally because they do not have enough energy.

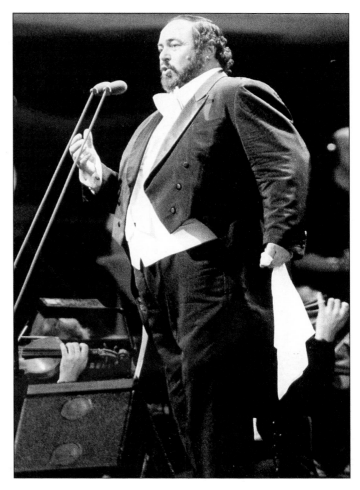

ABOVE Opera singer, Luciano Pavarotti, is able to sustain very long notes because he has learnt to fill his lungs totally with air between musical phrases. By breathing from his diaphragm he makes his lungs work more efficiently.

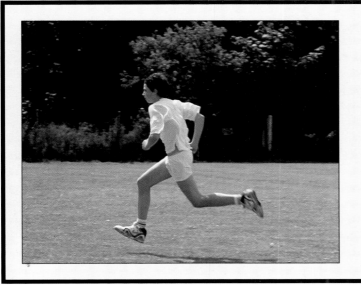

CHECKING YOUR BREATHING

Using the second hand of your watch or a stop-watch, count the number of times you breathe in a minute when you are sitting still doing nothing. Then take some steady exercise that you know you can keep up for about fifteen minutes. Stop every five minutes and measure your breathing rate. Then measure your breathing rate when you stop exercising and every three minutes for the next fifteen minutes.

See how high your breathing rate goes when it reaches a maximum, and how quickly it returns to normal after you stop your exercise. The sooner you are breathing normally, the fitter you are.

THE BRAIN AND BREATHING

Your brain can't just guess when to tell you to breathe in and out. It has to be told when you need oxygen. This job is done by receptors in the walls of some of your blood vessels. Just as the dipstick in the engine of a car will tell you when you are running low on oil, so these receptors tell the brain when levels of carbon dioxide are getting too high. A warning signal is sent to the breathing centre in the brain. This then sends messages down the nerves to the lungs and the diaphragm telling them that it's time to breathe in some more air so that the oxygen supply to the rest of the body is increased.

As the lungs expand, a second set of receptors, in the bronchioles and alveoli, go into action. These are called stretch receptors and it's their job to send messages to the brain when the lungs are full of air. The brain realizes that enough air has been breathed in and sends messages back to the lungs and diaphragm telling them to relax so that you can breathe out.

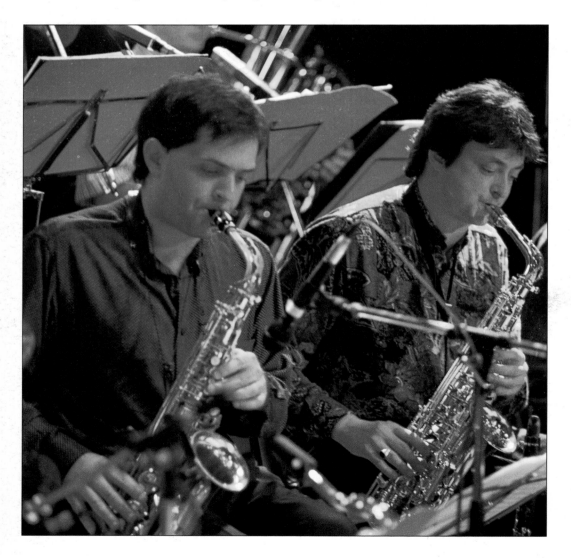

LEFT Playing a wind or brass instrument requires very efficient breathing and expert timing.

RIGHT This little boy makes it look so easy! But swimming underwater requires careful control over your breathing.

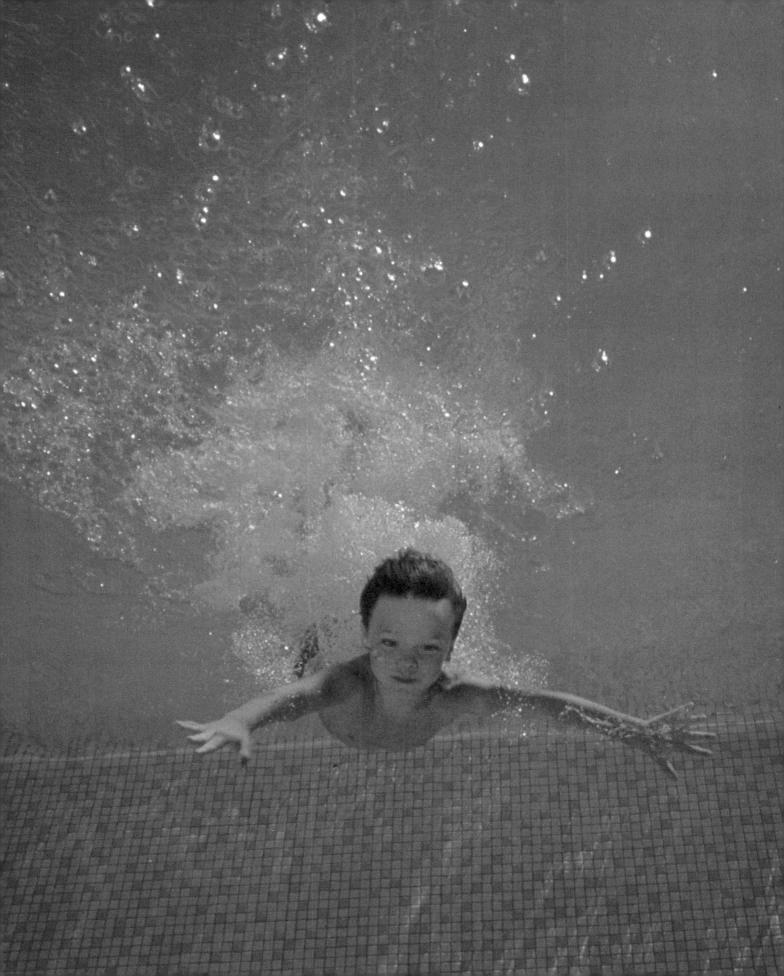

Most of the time you won't even be aware that you are breathing in and out. Your lungs just work automatically. Your brain will tell them when to inflate and when to deflate, without you having to think about it.

Sometimes you may want to take over the breathing. If you are at the seaside, for example, you may want to take lots of deep breaths of fresh air. Or if you are diving you may want to hold your breath.

You can do all of these things and your brain will gladly oblige by telling your lungs to adapt their breathing pattern. But if you deliberately breathe too fast - hyperventilate - you will confuse the whole system.

As you breathe harder and harder you will breathe out more and more carbon dioxide, so levels in your bloodstream will go down. Your receptors - not sensing much carbon dioxide - will not tell your brain that you need to breathe. You will stop breathing and the lack of carbon dioxide in your blood will make it more alkaline. This will make your muscles go into spasm.

This is what happens during mass hysteria. Hysteria makes people hyperventilate. They fall to the ground twitching and gasping as their brains try to make sense of the signals they are receiving. Hyperventilation can be counteracted by breathing into a paper (not plastic) bag.

COT DEATHS

Each year about 2,000 babies die as a result of 'cot death'. They seem healthy when they go to bed at night. But they are found dead in the morning. No one knows quite why this happens. But it has been shown that some babies stop breathing for quite long periods of time when they are asleep. There must be something wrong with the mechanism that should tell their brains when they need to breathe. In some cases, they do not start breathing again without help. Babies known to be at risk can be fitted with special alarms so their parents can be woken. Parents are also advised to lay their baby on his or her back when sleeping.

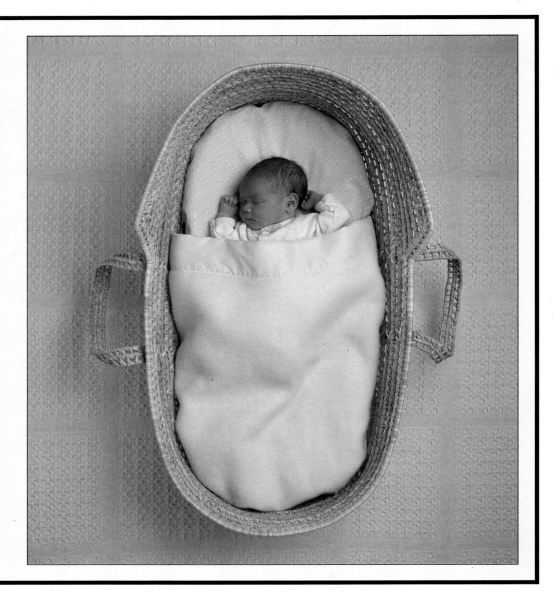

THE NOSE

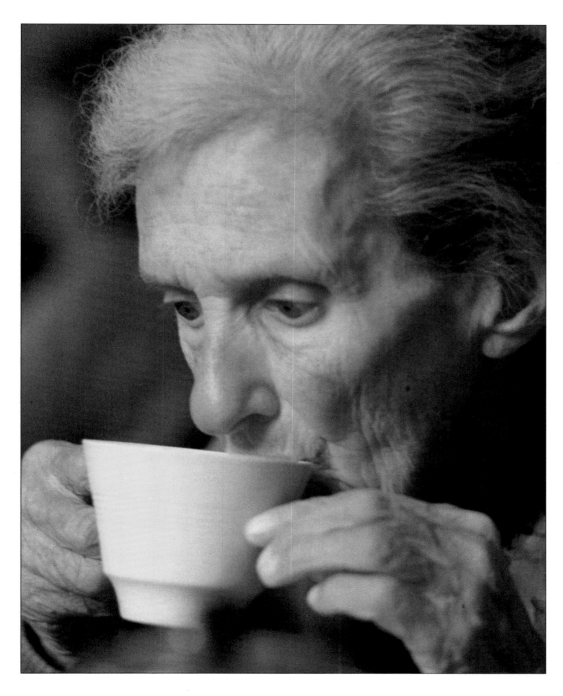

We don't just use our noses to smell things. Before it reaches the lungs, the air we breathe has been through the quality control system in our nose where it has been cleaned, warmed and given the 'all clear'.

The nose acts as a filter and heating system for the lungs. Hairs in the nostrils trap dirt in the air and prevent it from going down into the lungs. Cells in the lining of the nose produce sticky mucus which captures any particles that have escaped the hairs. Then, as the air goes up the nose, warmth from the blood in the tiny blood vessels in the nose helps to raise the temperature of the air.

Inside the bones around the bridge of the nose are four sets of air-filled cavities called sinuses. These also produce mucus and help prepare the air for its journey down to the lungs.

When you have a cold, the inside of your nose becomes swollen and vast amounts of mucus are produced. This is the nose's way of defending itself from attack by the germs that cause colds. But it is very uncomfortable for us.

A growing number of people have an 'allergic' nose. Their noses respond in the same way to harmless things in the air, such as pollen, dust and animal fur, as they do to germs. They become red and swollen and 'bunged up' with lots of mucus.

If nothing is done, the mucus can fill and eventually block the sinuses. This can happen after a cold or because of an allergy. If mucus is trapped in the sinuses for a long time it can become infected. Blocked sinuses can be very painful. Sufferers ache around their eyes and sometimes across much of their faces.

If you know someone who seems to have a cold all the time, they may well have an allergic nose. If they are worse in summer they are probably suffering from hay fever. And if they complain of being permanently bunged up, it is possible that they have sinusitis.

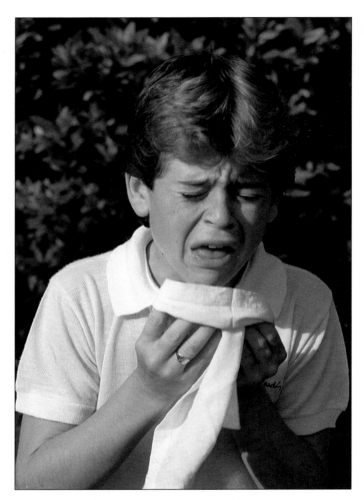

ABOVE Hay fever can make you pretty miserable. But there are tablets and sprays that can help stop your nose running.

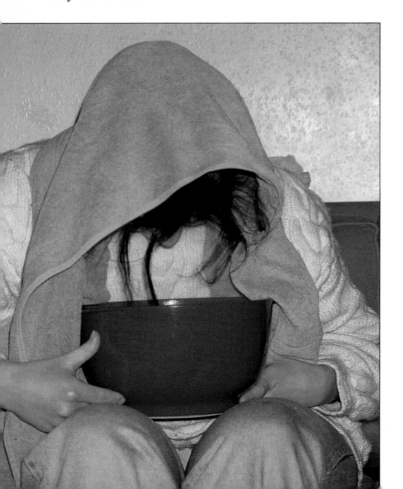

LEFT Inhaling steam is an old remedy for a blocked nose. But it can be quite effective. The towel stops the steam escaping.

UNBLOCKING NOSES

Sometimes blowing your nose is all you need to do to get rid of mucus. But if you feel very bunged up there are other simple remedies. Nose drops may stop the swelling in the nose or dry up some of the mucus. Steam treatment can also make your nose less blocked-up.

COLDS AND FLU

Each time you sneeze you spray the air around you with thousands of droplets of saliva and mucus. If you have a cold or flu the droplets will contain the germs that cause those infections and you'll pass them on to other people.

A cold can be caused by any one of 200 different viruses. There are fewer flu viruses, but year by year they are able to change slightly, so they can be even more of a nuisance than cold viruses. Some of them can make you feel terrible!

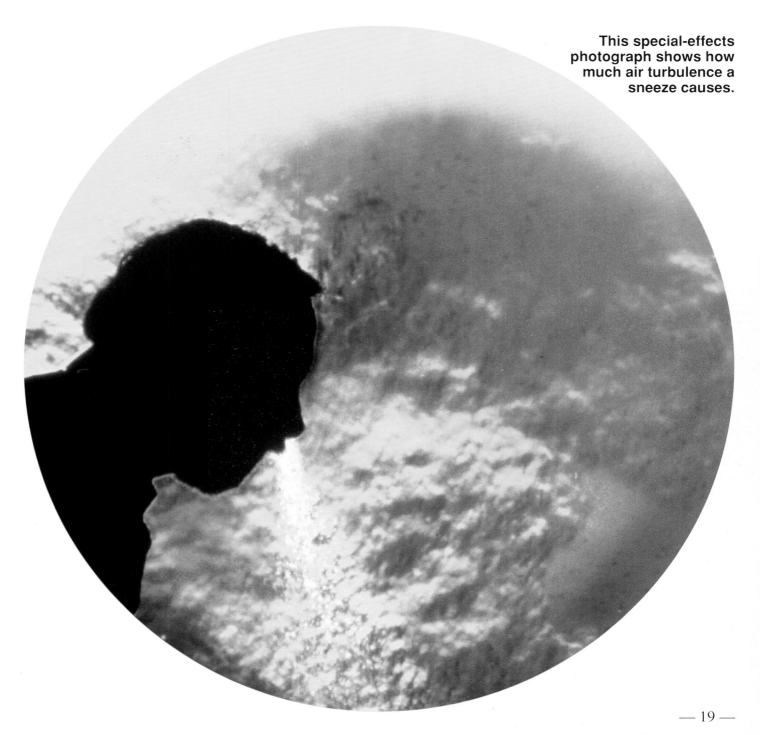

This special-effects photograph shows how much air turbulence a sneeze causes.

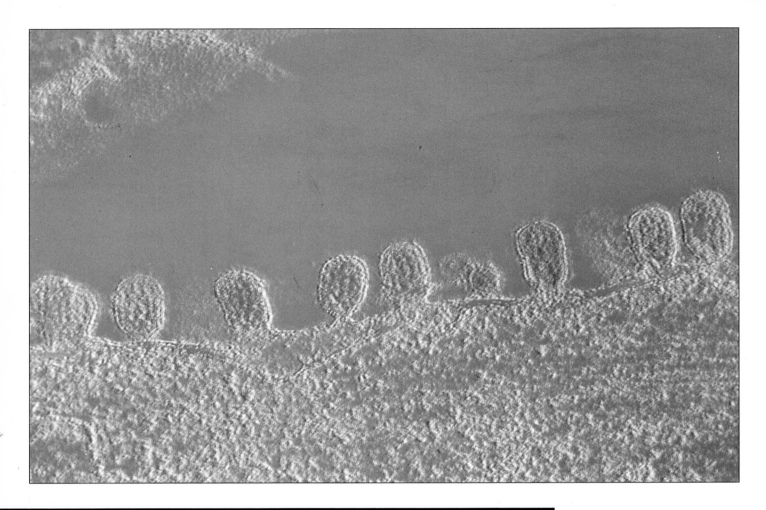

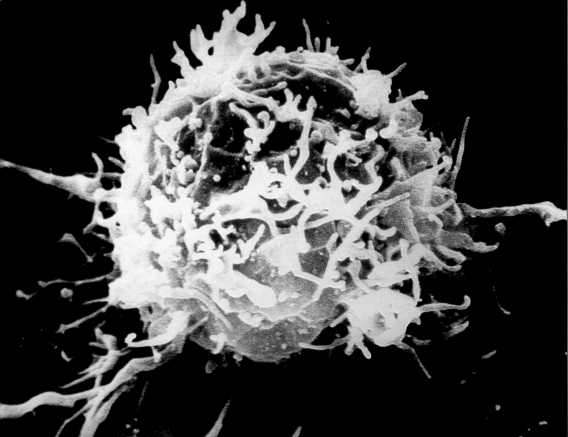

ABOVE This picture has had colour added to show particles of flu virus sitting on the surface of a cell, preparing to invade nearby cells.

LEFT This T-lymphocyte is the type of white blood cell which stands between you and nasty infections. But its spiky appearance won't be enough to scare off bacteria and viruses. It will need help from other immune cells.

Viruses are so tiny that you can't see any of them – not even through a typical school microscope. In fact, a bacterium is fifty times larger. A virus does not have its own cell to live in. It just consists of a piece of genetic material - DNA or RNA - and an outer coating of protein.

Cold and flu viruses spend most of their time invading human cells. When you breathe in virus-containing droplets, the viruses quickly get into the cells of your nose. They head for the nucleus in the centre of your cells where your own DNA is. Here, they quickly multiply and move on to attack the next cell.

Your body responds by activating your natural defences - your immune system. First on the scene are the white blood cells. They attack the viruses and produce proteins called antibodies. These antibodies not only attack viruses but also call in other cells to attack them too. With all this activity, the lining of your nose becomes swollen and you need lots of paper tissues as you produce large quantities of mucus.

Over the next few days a fierce battle is fought inside your nose and probably your throat. Eventually, the cold or flu virus loses and your own cells win.

If you have flu, the battle will probably spread further down, into your trachea and bronchi, and take longer to win. Your body temperature will rise and your head, your arms and your legs may ache. Scientists aren't sure whether the rise in temperature is part of the body's defence plan aimed at making life too hot for the viruses, or the result of the viral attack.

IN SEARCH OF A CURE

There is no cure for either a cold or flu. Painkillers will help relieve the aches and pains and bring your temperature down. Decongestants will help to unblock your nose. But scientists have not yet found any drugs that are effective against cold and flu viruses.

Antibiotic drugs are unlikely to do any good. They are designed to attack bacteria and, as you have seen, colds and flu are caused by viruses. The only time they may be helpful is for people, such as the elderly and those with long-term illnesses, who are at risk of getting a bacterial infection on top of their cold or flu.

There's no cure for flu. You just have to wait it out until your immune cells get the better of the virus.

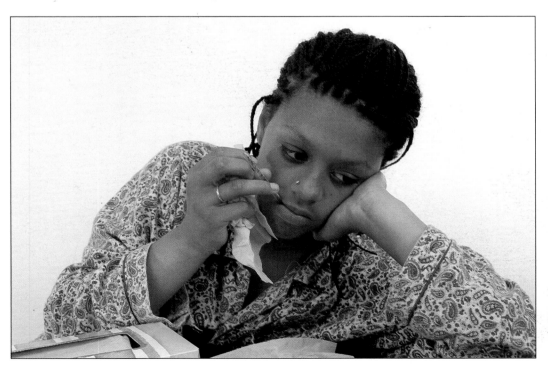

SMOKING

The list of chest diseases caused by smoking is long and unpleasant: lung cancer, emphysema, bronchitis, mouth cancer, cancer of the larynx... Many die slow, painful deaths. They aren't all old. They are men and women of all ages.

People who smoke are very stupid. Even if their smoking does not kill them it damages their lungs. They get more chest infections, they cough, wheeze and choke. They aren't able to run as far or as fast as they should because there isn't enough oxygen going to their cells. Their breath smells and their teeth decay. And when they blow smoke over their friends they can make them ill too. In fact, some non-smokers die because they have breathed in the cigarette fumes of their so-called friends over many years.

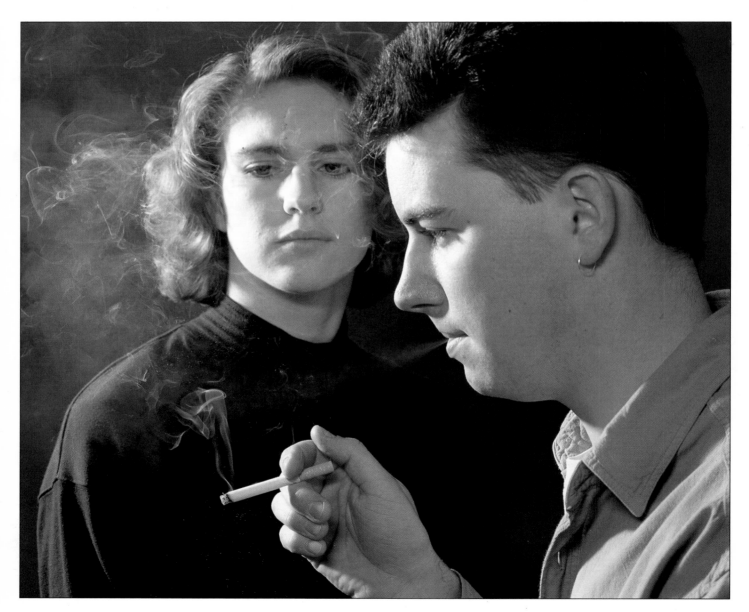

He's not just wrecking his lungs. He's damaging her health too.

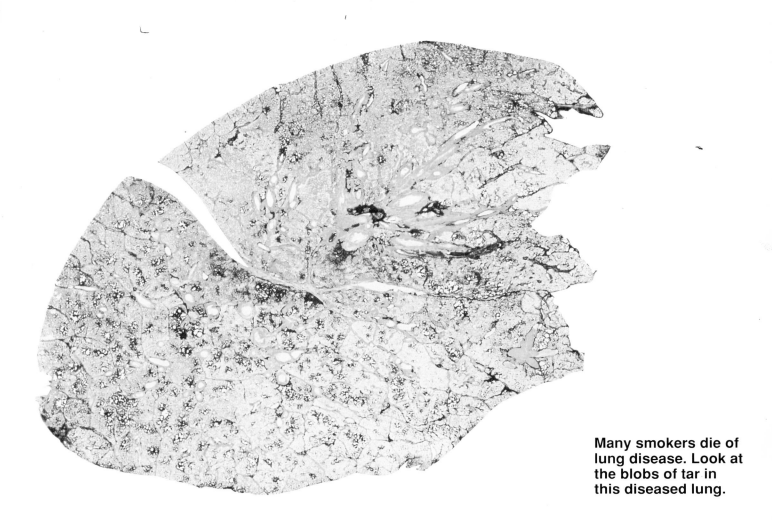

Many smokers die of lung disease. Look at the blobs of tar in this diseased lung.

Tobacco contains hundreds of chemicals. Some cause cancer. Others destroy the fragile walls of the bronchioles and the alveoli. One - carbon monoxide - pushes oxygen off the haemoglobin in the blood so that cells all over the body are starved of oxygen.

The nicotine in cigarettes is very addictive. Smokers get a physical and mental need for nicotine which only another cigarette can satisfy. If you saw inside a smoker's lungs you'd probably be sick. You'd find dead and dying cells, globules of blackened mucus waiting to be coughed up, shrivelled alveoli, scarred bronchioles and blocked and broken blood vessels.

Yet, each year thousands of young people start smoking. Once they are hooked they find it very hard to give up. Many people want to give up and some manage. But they rarely lose the craving for a cigarette.

There is no 'safe' cigarette. High tar, medium tar, low tar - they can all kill people and give them lung diseases. Do you know anyone dying of lung disease? It's very frightening. So please don't be tempted to start smoking.

DEATH SMOKE

Smoking kills hundreds of thousands of people each year. In Britain alone, it's estimated to be about 115,000 – that's one death every five minutes. On average, a cigarette takes five and a half minutes off your life. Smoking causes four times as many premature deaths as all other avoidable risks put together, including road accidents, alcohol abuse, drugs and suicide.

If you stop smoking your risk of dying returns to that of a non-smoker within ten to fifteen years.

THE TOBACCO INDUSTRY

The tobacco industry spends millions of pounds a year advertising cigarettes, cigars and pipe tobacco, despite the fact that these can kill and injure people. If advertisements told drug addicts to share needles which would spread AIDS there would be uproar. Yet smoking kills far more people each year than AIDS. Similarly if supermarkets sold cyanide we'd be horrified. Yet newsagents sell cigarettes and they contain cyanide too.

Why do some governments let tobacco companies advertise? The answer is because they get a lot of money in taxes on cigarettes. The tobacco industry also employs a lot of people. Many would lose their jobs if cigarette sales fell dramatically as a result of a ban on advertising.

In spite of this, some countries, such as France, Italy and Portugal have decided that smoking is so bad for your health that they have agreed to ban tobacco advertising. Governments that are against a ban argue that people will still smoke even if advertising is banned. People start smoking for many different reasons, including pressure from friends or relatives to have a cigarette. Clearly, advertising is not the only reason.

But advertising must help sales or companies wouldn't spend all that money! Advertisements show smokers as strong, tough, successful people – they also appear to be very healthy. They suggest that if you smoke you will be successful, attractive, even desirable, too.

Although this cigarette advertisement aims to persuade you otherwise, there's not much pleasure in bad breath, gum disease and throat cancer.

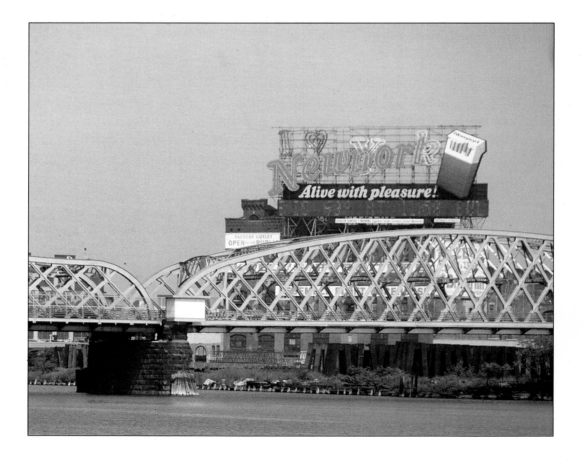

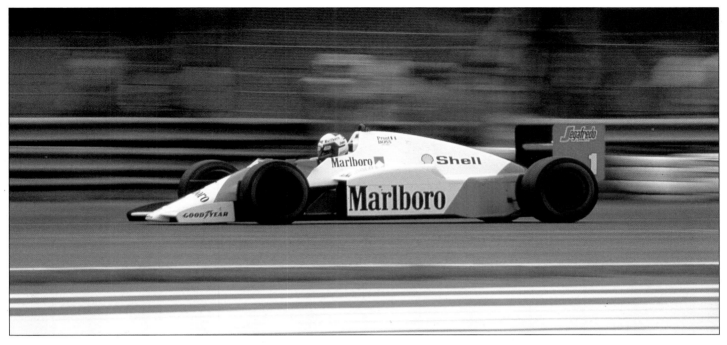

Cigarette advertising on a racing car. Whose life is at stake?

DEVELOPING COUNTRIES

In many countries advertising campaigns that promote smoking have been very successful. Recently the number of people who smoke in developing countries, such as India, China, Africa and South America, has shot up. About 70 per cent of Chinese men over twenty smoke and, between 2020 to 2025, an estimated 2 million Chinese people a year will die from smoking-related diseases such as lung cancer.

When they die we will be partly to blame. People in developing countries often follow the example of those in the West. Smoking is seen as a sign of wealth. So people who want to show their friends that they have money, buy cigarettes. Only by banning all tobacco advertising and reducing our smoking can we show people in poorer countries that it is a dangerous habit.

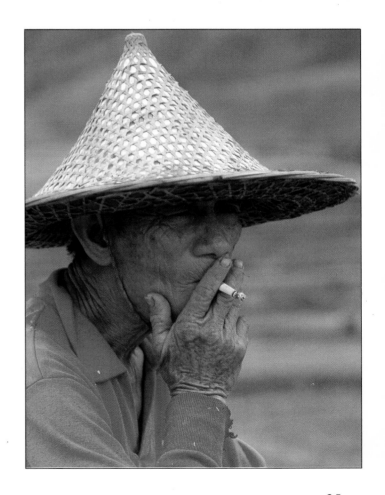

Who's to blame if this man dies of lung cancer? Is there anything we can do to help?

AIR POLLUTION

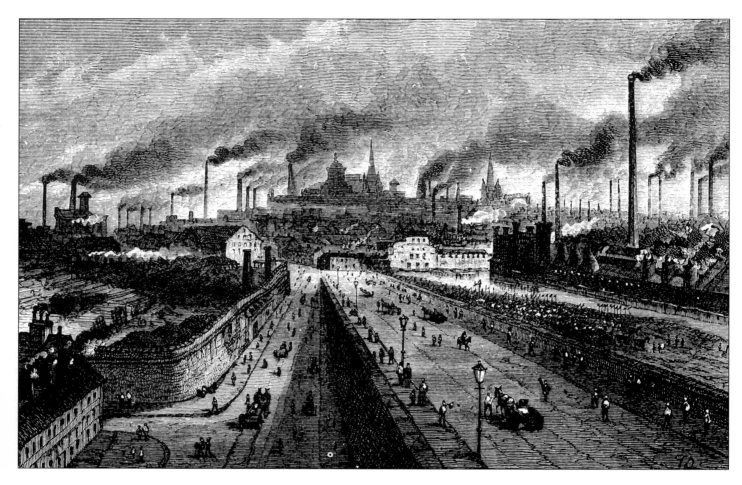

Not a car on the street but look at the pollution in the air over Sheffield in 1884.

Londoners called it a 'pea souper' – smog so thick you could barely see the person in front of you. It hung like a dirty cloud over the city. The smogs that covered big cities in the first half of this century came from levels of air pollution that would be unacceptable to us today. They were caused by the huge amounts of smoke from coal fires and factory chimneys.

Some cities still have smogs. But today they are caused by vehicle exhausts rather than coal fires. Los Angeles, Athens, Cairo, Bombay and Kuala Lumpur are just some of the cities whose sky-scrapers are often covered by smog.

Air pollution is not just ugly, it is dangerous to health. In 1952 smog hung over London for weeks and caused 4,000 deaths. The chemicals in smog attack the lungs. People who already have lung disorders such as bronchitis and asthma are at greatest risk. Even people with good lungs can feel breathless and uncomfortable when pollution levels are high.

Sulphur dioxide (SO_2) was the gas responsible for the London smogs of the 1950s. It is produced by power stations and diesel engines. In the lungs, it makes the bronchioles narrower so that less air can get in.

Sometimes smoke from coal fires mixes with sulphur dioxide. Smoke particles can get trapped in the lungs and cause damage, especially if they contain cancer-causing chemicals.

Nitrogen dioxide (NO2) is one of a family of chemicals called NOX (oxides of nitrogen). They are produced when fuel is burnt in cars and power stations. When they are breathed in they irritate the lining of the bronchioles and can make breathing more difficult.

In summer, sunlight can react with NOX and hydrocarbons (also found in car exhaust) to produce ozone. Ozone irritates the lungs and makes breathing more difficult for people with asthma and other lung diseases, or those who are exercising when ozone levels are high.

Carbon monoxide is another gas found in vehicle exhaust. In large amounts it prevents the blood from carrying oxygen around the body.

When nitrogen and sulphur dioxides in the air combine with water droplets they may form acid air, which also irritates the lungs. If they then fall to the ground as acid rain they can badly damage plants and trees.

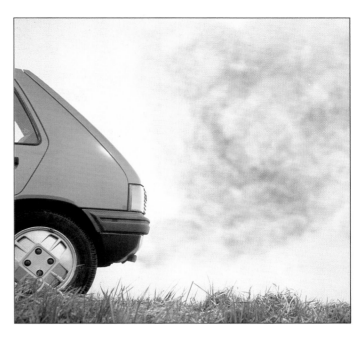

ABOVE It's hard to imagine life without cars. But we aren't helping the environment.

GAS MASKS

When you are exercising you breathe faster and harder to provide your muscles with enough oxygen. However, in busy town and city centres you also breathe in large amounts of pollution from the air.

You have probably seen some cyclists, motor-bike riders and joggers wearing gas masks to protect their lungs from polluted air (right). Some of these are very effective in filtering out most of the chemicals such as NOX and SO2 that upset the lungs.

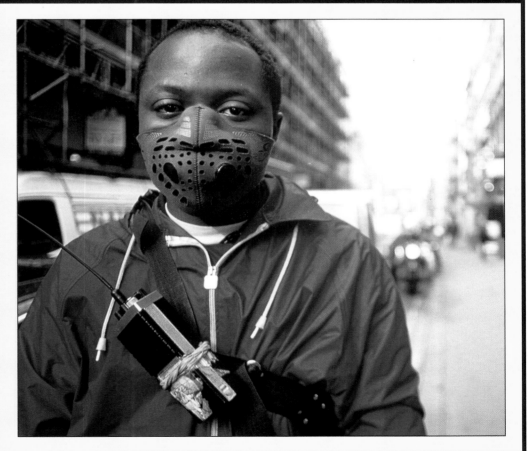

AIR-CONDITIONING

Living and working in modern air-conditioned buildings can make us ill. More and more people wheeze, sneeze, have headaches, sore eyes, itchy skin and feel generally unwell because of the lack of fresh air in some buildings. It's called 'sick building syndrome'.

There are several reasons why this happens. Microbes can live in air-conditioning ducts and may go round and round a building. So bacterial and viral infections are passed to everyone in an office. Central heating means that buildings are kept much warmer and drier than they used to be and many bugs like this.

It isn't just offices that can be 'sick'. Our homes may also harbour creatures that make us ill. Thick carpets instead of wooden floors attract dust mites.

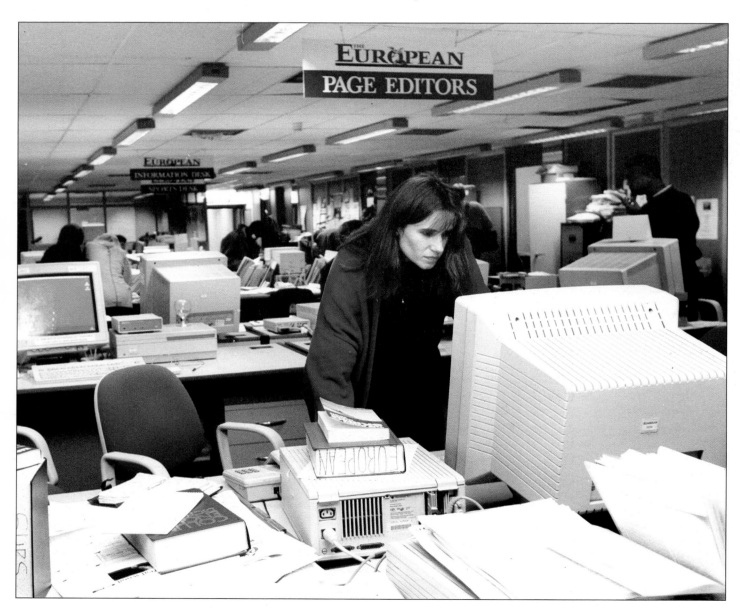

A modern air-conditioned office provides a good home for many germs.

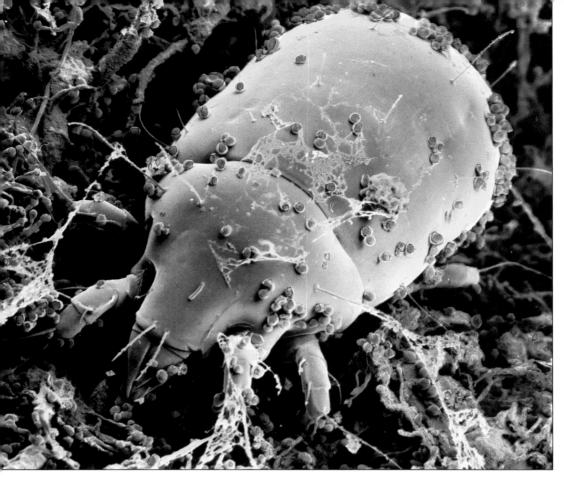

The house dust mite isn't really green. Colour has been added to make it stand out. There are millions of mites in your bed, your chairs, your carpets, and your curtains – but you won't be able to see them without a microscope!

BELOW Animal fur is one of the most common causes of asthma.

These tiny little mites are related to spiders and they are found anywhere that is warm and cosy. That means carpets, chair covers, curtains and bedding. There is a protein in their faeces which makes some people wheeze and have a runny nose. In fact, more people are thought to be allergic to house dust mites than anything else.

Experts advise us to open windows and reduce the humidity of our homes - even in winter. Carpets need to be cleaned regularly and bedding washed at high temperatures to kill dust mites. If that doesn't work it may be best to pull up carpets and put down hard floors with rugs that can easily be taken up and shaken.

OTHER ALLERGIES

Pollen and animal fur are the other two things most likely to upset the noses and lungs of people who are allergic to them. Trying to avoid them is easier said than done! But it is the best way of reducing the risk of hay fever or asthma.

If you know you are allergic to animal fur you shouldn't really get a pet. If you already have one, at least keep it out of your bedroom and off the furniture. Don't touch your face when you are playing with your pet and always wash your hands after you've been playing with it.

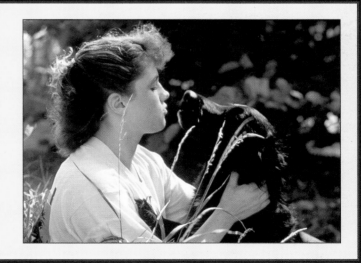

CHEST DISORDERS

Sometimes a cold or a bout of flu can go 'on to your chest'. This means that the infection has spread down into the smaller airways in your lungs and made them inflamed and sore. This is called acute bronchitis.

Some people - mostly smokers - have inflamed airways for many months at a time, especially through the winter. This is called chronic bronchitis. It may have started with a cold or flu or the chemicals in their cigarette smoke may have made their airways inflamed and full of mucus. Sufferers feel very run down.

Pneumonia is an infection in the alveoli. They become clogged with fluid and cells and unable to absorb oxygen normally. Young and fit people usually get over pneumonia with antibiotics.

But it can kill frail elderly people, especially those who are bed-bound after a serious stroke or cancer.

Pneumonia is usually caused by a bacterium. That's why antibiotics are so effective. But sometimes it is caused by a virus and is harder to treat.

Emphysema is also a disease of the alveoli. Once again, most cases are caused by smoking but some people have an inherited disorder that makes them prone to the disease. The alveoli become permanently damaged and unable to provide the body with enough oxygen. Drugs can help but many people with emphysema need extra oxygen.

There is no doubt that people who smoke are more likely to have chronic bronchitis and emphysema - often both. They are very unpleasant diseases. Sufferers cough, and are nearly always breathless. In the later stages of the diseases they are too breathless even to stand up.

LEGIONNAIRE'S DISEASE

In 1976, a group of former soldiers (members of the American Legion) were struck down by severe pneumonia. The type of bacterium which caused the outbreak was called Legionella and all outbreaks which have happened since have been called Legionnaire's Disease. Like other forms of pneumonia, it responds to antibiotics but is more serious in old people.

Legionnaire's Disease is not spread from person to person but is caught by breathing infected water droplets from air-conditioning systems. Each outbreak attracts a lot of publicity because people get frightened that the bacterium may be in their air pipes too.

These are the bacteria which cause Legionnaire's Disease – a kind of pneumonia.

RIGHT The X-ray of a chest showing pneumonia in the right lung.

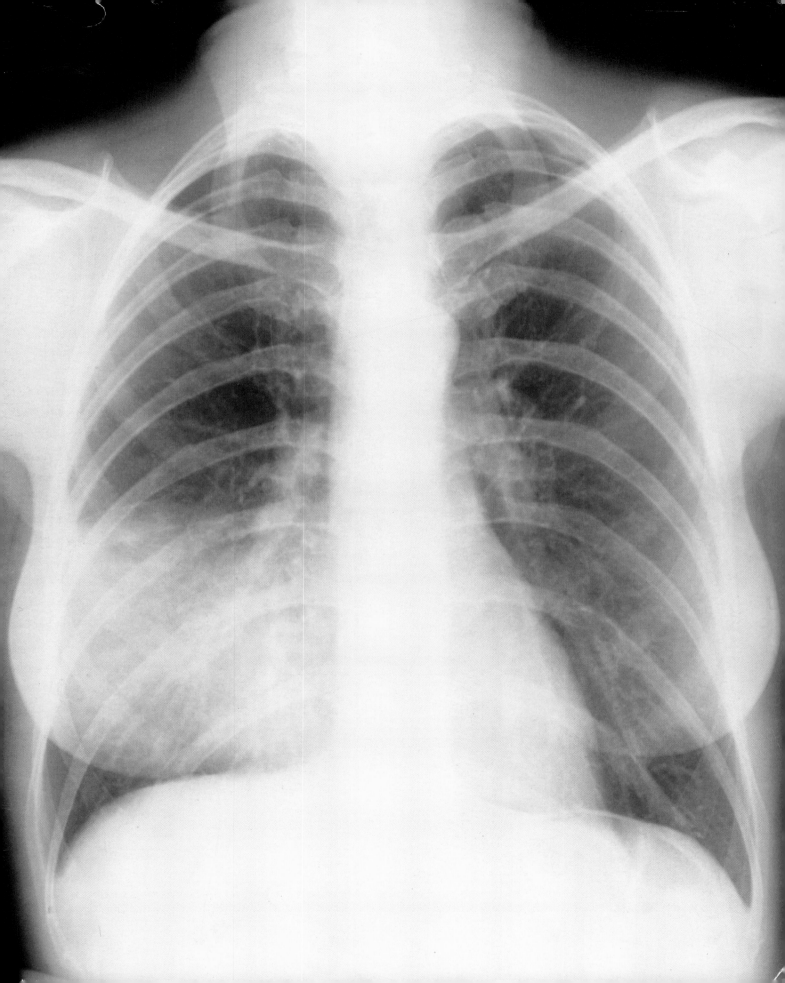

ASTHMA

One in ten children has asthma. The muscles in the walls of their airways contract when they shouldn't. Their tubes get narrower so less air can get in and out of the lungs. Their alveoli are working as hard as they can. But there simply isn't enough air for them to process.

As carbon dioxide begins to build up in the blood, the brain sends signals to the lungs to breathe faster. They try, but they still can't satisfy the body's needs. Breathing becomes very inefficient - lots of quick, shallow, noisy breaths. This noise is called wheezing.

There are several reasons why the muscles in the airways contract and cause an asthma attack. Many asthmatics are 'allergic' to things in the air. Their immune systems, which normally protect them from infection, over-react to harmless things like pollen, dust and animal fur. These immune cells set off a chain of events which results in the airways getting narrower.

Some asthmatics even over-react to things like cold air or cigarette smoke. Their airways immediately seize up and they start to wheeze.

Luckily, asthma doesn't have to stop you doing the things you want to. Cricketer Ian Botham and Olympic swimmer Adrian Moorhouse are just two of many sports people who have reached the top despite their asthma. There are plenty of successful business people, actors, doctors and dancers who also have asthma. This is because there are plenty of very effective drugs that can be taken to open up airways and stop wheezing or prevent the immune system from over-reacting to things in the first place.

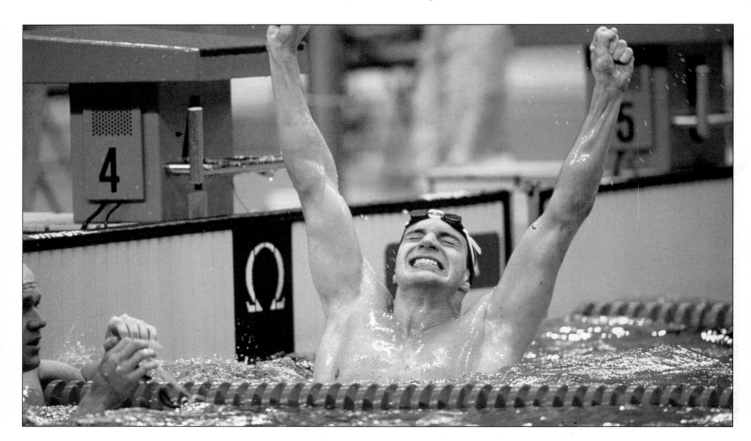

Olympic swimmer Adrian Moorhouse shows that asthma hasn't stopped him!

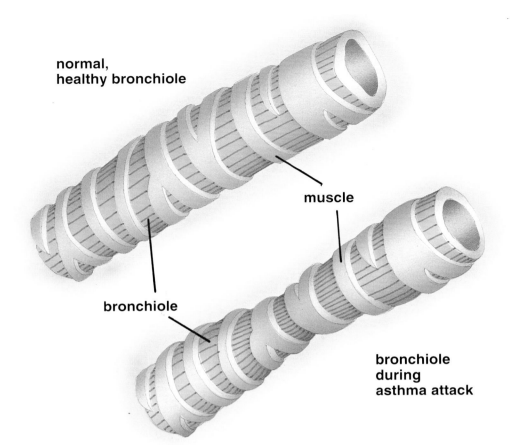

normal,
healthy bronchiole

LEFT In asthma,
muscle wrapped
around the
bronchioles
contracts, narrowing
the airway and
restricting air flow so
it becomes hard to
breathe.

muscle

bronchiole

bronchiole
during
asthma attack

BELOW A quick puff
with her inhaler and
this girl will soon be
able to play with her
friends again.

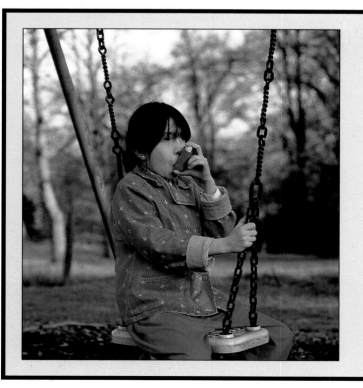

INHALED STEROIDS

Most asthma experts now believe that it is
important not just to relieve asthma
symptoms when they happen but to get at
the cause. When the immune cells see
something they don't like they don't just
make the airways close up. The airways also
become inflamed and too much mucus is
produced. This can go on for a long time and,
eventually, it will leave scars on the walls of
the airways.

It is now possible to take drugs that damp
down this inflammation. They are called
steroids. You can inhale them straight into
the lungs - just like other drugs that make the
airways wider.

Some people do worry about taking
steroids. But when they are inhaled they are
very unlikely to cause any problems. And
they are very effective at preventing the
airways from becoming inflamed.

TUBERCULOSIS

Before drugs were discovered that could kill TB bacteria, people believed in 'touching' by Kings as a form of treatment. Charles II (pictured here in a drawing from 1654) had a particularly good reputation.

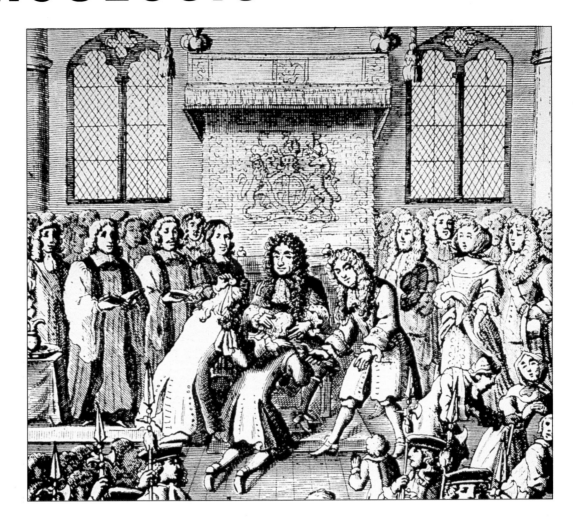

Tuberculosis (TB) was the scourge of the eighteenth and nineteenth centuries and the first half of the twentieth century. Every year, millions of people worldwide died of the dreaded disease. No family was left untouched. In 1882, the German scientist Robert Koch discovered microbes in the lungs of people with TB. But it wasn't until the early 1950s that drugs were discovered that could kill the bacteria and save many lives.

Before that, fresh air and rest were the main treatments. Men and women with TB were sent to hospitals in the Alps and other mountain regions where the air was believed to be cleaner.

The bacterium which causes TB can attack any organ of the body but the lungs are its usual target.

The microbe gets into the lungs and is soon surrounded by immune cells trying to destroy it. This mixture of bacterial and human cells is called a tubercle. Tubercles join together and some of the lung tissue caught in the middle dies. Sometimes the lung heals but, without treatment, large areas may be destroyed. This can be fatal.

Modern drugs can stop the TB microbe in its tracks. In the 1950s and 1960s doctors in mobile vans X-rayed thousands of people to find those infected with TB so that they could receive the new treatment. And schoolchildren started to be immunized (given injections) against the bacterium. As a result, TB is rare in developed countries but is still widespread in developing countries.

PREVENTING INFECTION

TB is still found in some 'western' countries among people in Asian and African communities. They were infected with the bacterium before they left their own countries and can pass it on to their families and friends. It is important that they are found quickly before too much lung damage is done. The infection can be treated easily and effectively with drugs. Those people who are not infected can be immunized (given an injection) against the micro-organism that causes TB.

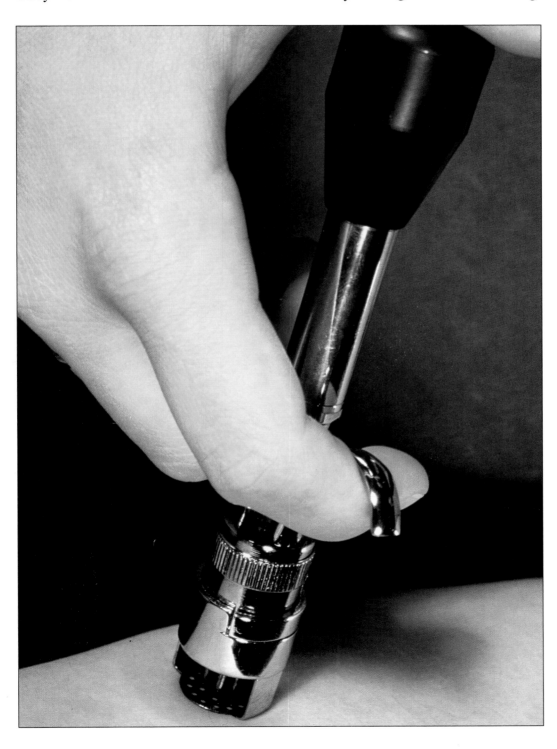

Today, children are routinely immunized (given an injection as protection) against TB. First, they are tested to see if they have any immunity to the bacterium (as in the picture). If they don't, they are given the vaccine.

CYSTIC FIBROSIS

Cystic fibrosis is the most common serious inherited disease. Children with cystic fibrosis produce too much mucus in their lungs and most lack important enzymes that they need to be able to digest their food. The extra mucus makes them prone to serious chest infections.

Each of our cells contains all the genetic material - DNA - which controls what we look like and what sort of person we are. But some of these genes may be faulty. We inherit two copies of most of our genes - one from each parent. Children who inherit a cystic fibrosis gene from one of their parents will not get the disease. But they may pass it on to their children. One in twenty-five people is a carrier of the abnormal gene which causes cystic fibrosis. Only children who inherit the bad gene from both their parents get the disease.

Good drugs and regular physiotherapy to get rid of some of the mucus have meant that people with cystic fibrosis do much better now than even ten years ago. They can also take digestive enzymes to replace those that are missing. And, at the first sign of a chest infection, they can have antibiotics.

Some children with cystic fibrosis have had heart and lung transplants to replace their diseased lungs. It is easier to transplant the lungs and heart together than just the lungs. So the healthy heart of the cystic fibrosis patient can be given to someone else who just needs a heart.

Children who have had transplants do very well. They still need their extra digestive enzymes but their new lungs are normal. All of those who have had the operation are being carefully checked to see how they get on as they grow up.

Daily physiotherapy for a girl with cystic fibrosis helps to dislodge the mucus in her lungs so she can cough it up. There is then less chance of her lungs becoming infected.

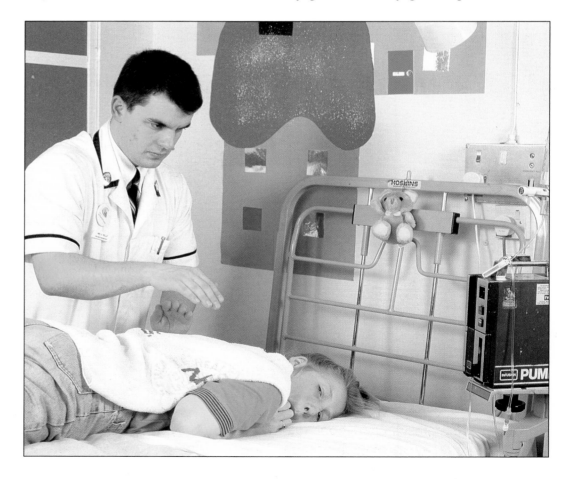

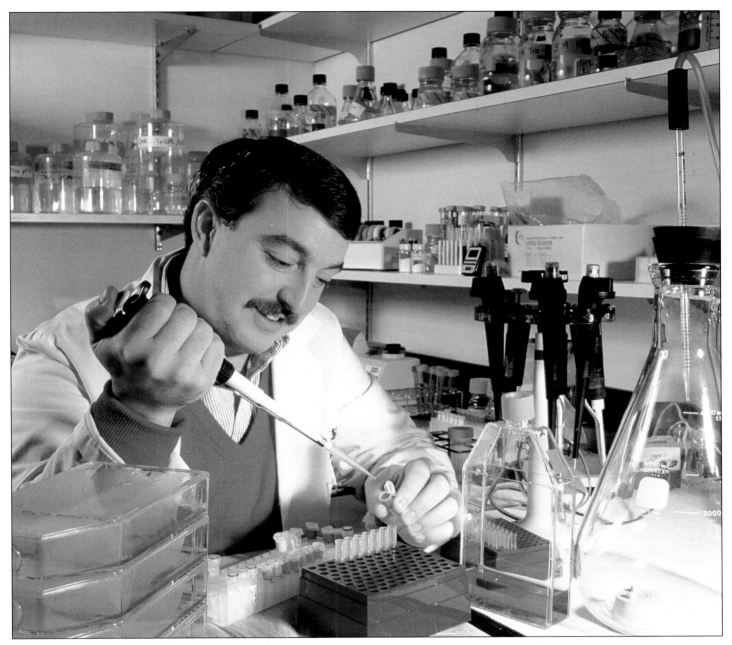

A gene therapist at work in his laboratory.

FINDING THE GENE

The gene that causes cystic fibrosis was discovered in 1989. It wouldn't have been possible without the scientific advances of the last ten years. In the end, researchers hope to find out the job of all 50,000 genes in each of our cells.

If they know what they should do they may be able to treat them so that they all work properly. This is called gene therapy. A few people have already had gene therapy for very severe diseases of the immune system and, before long, doctors could be using gene therapy to treat diseases such as cystic fibrosis. In the meantime they will continue to use a combination of drugs, physiotherapy, enzymes and transplants.

ANAESTHETIC GASES

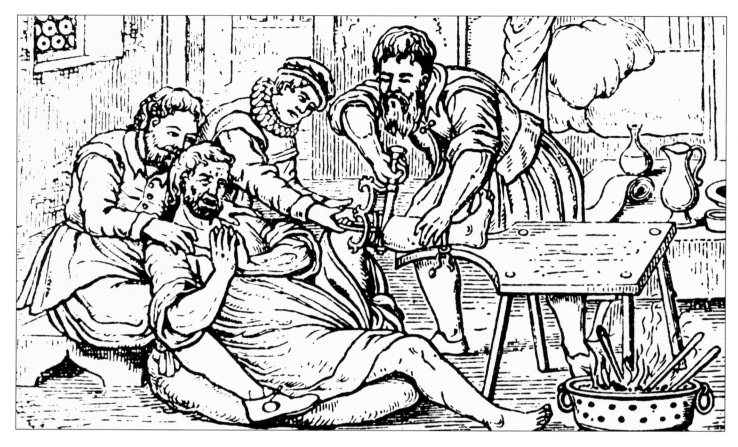

Before the days of anaesthetics, operations could be extremely painful.

It's hard to imagine having an operation without an anaesthetic to get rid of the pain. But, until the middle of the nineteenth century, that's exactly what happened. Operations were carried out as quickly as possible so that patients weren't in pain for too long.

In 1844, nitrous oxide (N20) was the first gas to be used successfully as an anaesthetic during the removal of a tooth. It is still widely used today with oxygen, to keep people asleep during surgical operations.

Gases like nitrous oxide and, later, ether, chloroform and halothane, could only be used once doctors understood how the lungs worked. During the eighteenth century they began to understand what happens to the air that we breathe in.

Before it was used as an anaesthetic, nitrous oxide was used as a social drug, much like alcohol today. It was called laughing gas because when people breathed it in they felt much happier and started to laugh. They did not - as happens in *Mary Poppins* - end up on the ceiling when they inhaled the gas. But they did feel much better.

In 1846, ether was the first gas to be used in a major operation - to remove a tumour. But ether catches fire easily and people who breathe it in are very sick when they wake up from their operation. So doctors looked for other drugs that had fewer unpleasant side effects.

Today, halothane and nitrous oxide are probably the most widely used anaesthetic gases. They don't, of course, put you to sleep by working on the lungs. They get into the blood, via the alveoli, and are transported around the body to parts of the brain that control consciousness.

Usually, anaesthetic gases are used with other anaesthetic drugs that are injected directly into the bloodstream. This is because doctors have found that if they use several different drugs they can use less of each one. So people wake up more quickly after their operations and are able to get up and about sooner.

In fact, many operations are now done under local anaesthetic. This means that the patient stays awake but feels no pain.

ANAESTHETICS IN CHILDBIRTH

We have Queen Victoria to thank for making the use of anaesthetics in childbirth acceptable. She used chloroform to get her through the birth of her son Prince Leopold in 1853. Ever since, women have been able to have drugs to relieve the pain of having a baby.

Some choose a mixture of nitrous oxide and oxygen while others have drugs that are injected into their bloodstream.

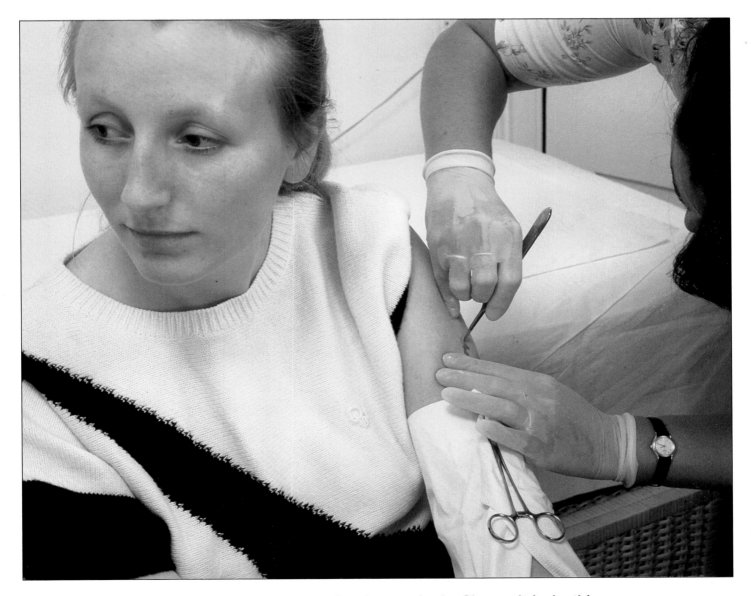

This woman is having a wart removed under local anaesthetic. She can't feel a thing.

ARTIFICIAL VENTILATION

Each year, thousands of people owe their lives to a machine that acts as a pair of lungs for them. Premature babies, car accident victims and people who have had major operations are just some of those who need a ventilator. The alveoli in their lungs are able to absorb oxygen from the air and get rid of carbon dioxide. But, for some reason, the muscles in their chests are unable to make the lungs inflate and deflate so they can't inhale and exhale properly.

The muscles of tiny premature babies are simply too weak for them to breathe on their own. People who have been in car accidents or have had major operations may be so deeply unconscious that their brains stop sending messages to the muscles in their chests telling them to breathe.

The ventilator is a machine that breathes for you. A tube, which is attached to the ventilator, goes down through the mouth or nose and into the lungs. Air is then pumped down the tube to inflate the lungs and provide much needed oxygen.

The rate at which the lungs are inflated and deflated and the amounts of oxygen and carbon dioxide in the bloodstream are continuously monitored to be sure that the patient is getting the right amount of air.

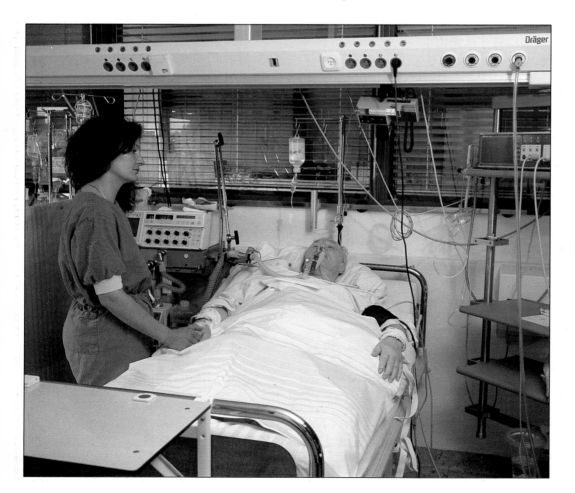

LEFT A ventilator keeps this man's lungs working while he recovers from a heart attack.

OPPOSITE The man at the back of the picture is lying in an iron lung to help him breathe. The woman in the wheelchair has a more advanced device which allows her to move around while her lungs are artificially ventilated.

People who need artificial ventilation are usually treated in the intensive care unit of a hospital. Some people remain unconscious - in a coma - for months. Ventilators can go on breathing for them all that time. Others gradually come out of their comas and start to breathe again for themselves.

Sometimes, it becomes clear that a person will never come out of their coma because their brain is too badly damaged. His or her relatives may then decide to switch off the ventilator so that he or she can die peacefully. Obviously this is a heart-rending decision to have to make.

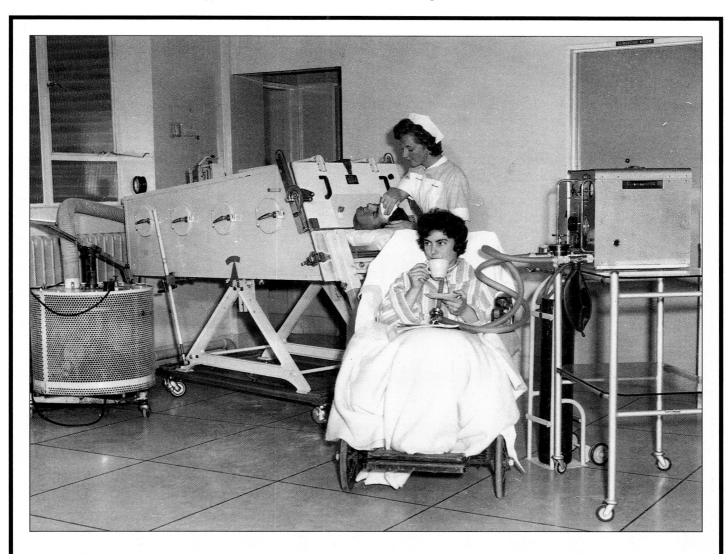

IRON LUNGS

Today's ventilators were developed from the original 'iron lungs' that were used to keep polio victims alive during the epidemic that occurred in the 1950s.

People with polio become paralysed and cannot move. In the worst cases, their chest muscles stop working. The iron lung was developed to make them breathe. Instead of air being pumped down into their lungs, their bodies were placed in large tanks with only their heads poking out. When air inside the tank was sucked out, their lungs inflated and air was taken in through their mouths. Air was then pumped back into the tanks so that the increased pressure on the outside of their chests pushed their lungs flat so that air was breathed out.

Fortunately, most of the people who survived polio were left only partly paralysed and, in the end, they were able to breathe again without their iron lungs.

BETTER BREATHING

How long can you hold your breath? Most people can do it for between thirty and fifty seconds. If you take several quick, deep breaths first, you will be able to hold your breath for longer. This is because the amount of carbon dioxide in your blood will go down. So it will be longer before your brain orders your lungs to inflate.

You can do this as a short experiment on dry land. But you should be careful about holding your breath under water. Some people have drowned because their brain allowed them to hold their breath for too long. They had too little oxygen in their blood and lost consciousness before they could get to the surface.

Some mammals, such as seals, can stay under water without taking a breath for up to fifteen minutes. But their red blood cells can carry more oxygen and, as they dive, their heart rate goes down and blood only goes to vital organs. So they need less oxygen.

If you go above about 3,050 metres you will notice that you get out of breath more easily. You may even feel sick and dizzy. This is because there is less oxygen in the air at this level than there is nearer sea level.

As the body tries to make up for the shortfall you breathe more quickly. This has precisely the wrong effect. By breathing faster the amount of carbon dioxide in your blood falls and your brain thinks you do not need to breathe. You soon feel very ill.

People who go higher and higher without waiting for their bodies to get used to the altitude become very sick and may even die. What they should do is spend a few days at the higher altitude and wait for their bodies to get used to the air. After a few days the bone marrow will start producing more red blood cells so more oxygen can be carried around the body.

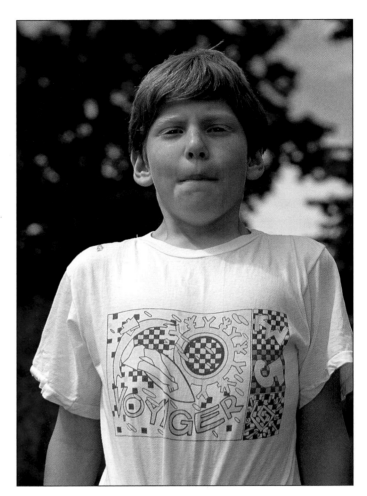

How long do you think this boy will be able to hold his breath? About thirty seconds? Be careful when holding your breath – it can be quite dangerous!

Athletes who want to perform better train at a high altitude so that they can carry more oxygen in their blood. If their competition is at sea-level - with normal amounts of oxygen in the air - they will then be at an advantage because they can get extra oxygen to their muscles. This means they can move faster and keep going for longer.

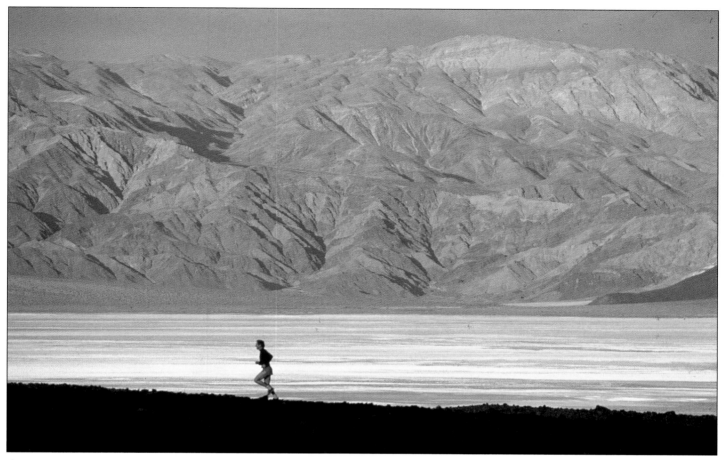

Altitude training can help improve an athlete's performance on the big day.

WHAT TO DO IF SOMEONE STOPS BREATHING

If you are with someone, send them to fetch help.

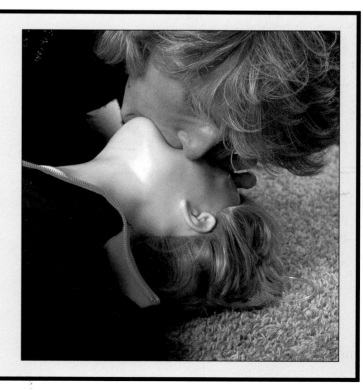

● To help someone to breathe, turn him or her on to their back. Tip the head back, open the mouth and check that there is nothing blocking the throat. Pinch the nose shut. Take a deep breath and place your mouth over his or hers. Blow strongly into the lungs.

● Take another deep breath and breathe out into his or her lungs. Keep doing this every five seconds. Between each breath listen for air coming out of the person's mouth and watch the chest fall. Go on breathing into the mouth until he or she starts to breathe again or help arrives.

DOES ALL LIFE NEED OXYGEN?

It's impossible for us to imagine life without oxygen. If the oxygen supply to the brain stops for more than a few moments, cells start to die. Within two to three minutes the damage is irreversible.

You probably know that, on Earth, plants replace all the oxygen used up by animals. They convert carbon dioxide and water into carbohydrate and oxygen. The process is called photosynthesis. We don't know of any other planets that have enough oxygen for life as we know it. It is possible that there are other forms of life that don't need oxygen to live. But life on Earth has evolved over millions of years to use oxygen in its cells and we can't change that. Even small changes in the gases that we breathe can make us ill.

It is unlikely that we will ever 'run out' of oxygen. But levels of carbon dioxide and some pollutant gases in the air are rising. If this goes on, more people will suffer from lung diseases.

If we treat our lungs badly it is only ourselves who will suffer. But what we do to our air today will affect generations of people who live after us.

RIGHT The devastation caused by acid rain.

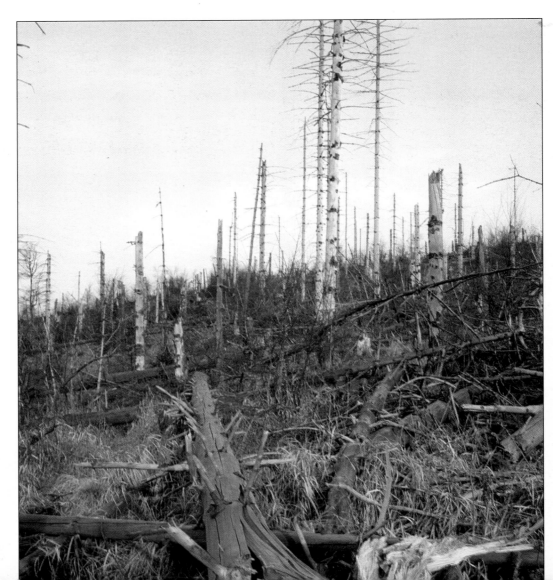

OPPOSITE Lush forest in the Malaysian jungle helps produce oxygen to sustain life on this planet.

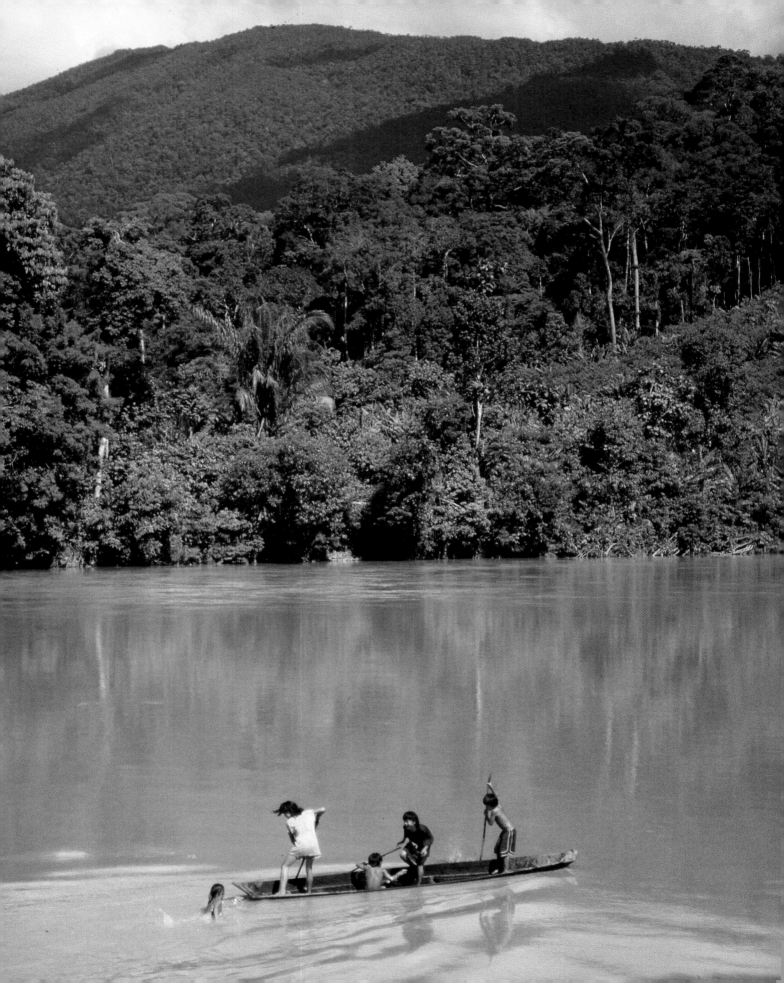

GLOSSARY

Allergy reaction of the immune system to a harmless substance that may cause wheezing and runny noses.

Alveoli tiny air sacs in the lung where oxygen is absorbed into the blood and carbon dioxide removed.

Antibiotic a drug that kills bacteria.

Bacterium a germ.

Bronchiole small airway in the lung that leads into an alveolus.

Bronchitis swelling of the bronchi or bronchioles caused by an infection or by irritant chemicals.

Bronchus one of two large airways that lead from the trachea into the lungs.

Capillary tiny blood vessel from which gases pass into and out of cells.

Cystic fibrosis serious inherited lung disease.

Diaphragm sheet of muscle below the lungs that is important for breathing.

Emphysema serious lung disease of the alveoli.

Haemoglobin red colouring in red blood cells that carries oxygen around the body.

Intercostal muscle between the ribs.

Larynx voice box.

NOX (oxides of nitrogen) pollutant chemicals in the air.

Pharynx throat.

Pneumonia serious infection of the lungs caused by a bacterium or a virus.

Surfactant slippery fluid in the airways which makes breathing easier.

Trachea tube that carries air from the throat to the bronchi.

Tuberculosis (TB) serious bacterial infection, usually of the lungs, which has been almost wiped out in developed countries.

Virus tiny germ that causes colds and flu and many other infections.

BOOKS TO READ

Let's Discuss Smoking by Vanora Leigh (Wayland, 1983)

Smoke Ring: The Politics of Tobacco by Peter Taylor (Bodley Head, 1984)

Acid Rain by Stephen Sterling (Wayland, 1991)

Atmosphere by John Baines (Wayland, 1991)

Smoking by Anne Charlish (Wayland, 1990)

Twentieth Century Medicine by Jenny Bryan (Wayland, 1988)

World Health by Janie Hampton (Wayland, 1987)

All About Health. An Introduction to Health Education by Dorothy Baldwin (OUP, 1985)

The Lungs and Breathing by Brian R. Ward (Franklin Watts, 1982)

ACKNOWLEDGEMENTS

All Sport 12 (Gary Mortimore), 32 (Tony Duffy), 43 (top, Ancil Nance); Chapel Studios 10, 21; Eye Ubiquitous 11 (top, Helene Rogers), 14 (Mostyn 92), 18 (bottom, Helene Rogers) 21 (Helene Rogers), 24 (T. Baverstock), 25 (bottom, Julia Waterlow), 42 (Yiorgus Nikiteas); Explorer 14; Life Science Images cover background; Mary Evans Picture Library 26; Planet Earth cover and title page; Reflections 13 (bottom, J. Woodcock); Science Photo Library 4 (CNRI), 5 (Peter Menzel), 7 (top, Biophoto Associates/bottom, Simon Fraser/Princess Mary Hospital, Newcastle), 8 (Dr Tony Brain), 9 (CNRI), 19 (Dr Gary Settles), 20 (top, CNRI/bottom NIBSC), 22 (Sheila Terry), 23 (James Stevenson), 27 (bottom, Jo Pasieka), 29 (top, CNRI), 30 (Barry Dowsett), 31, 33 (John Durham), 34 (Dr J. Burgess), 35 (Biophoto Associates), 36 (Simon Fraser/RVI, Newcastle-upon-Tyne), 37 (Will & Demi McIntyre), 38, 39 (Hattie Young), 43 (bottom, Blair Seitz); Skjold 10, 11 (bottom); The Environmental Picture Library 44 (Paul Glendell), 45 (C. Jones); Topham 13 (top), 17, 28, 41; WPL 10, 29 (bottom, Julia Davey); Zefa 6 (J. Feingersh), 11 (bottom, N. Schaefer), 13 (top and bottom), 15 (Pelegic Eye), 16, 18 (top), 25 (top), 27 (top, Dr. Mueller), 40.
Artwork: Malcolm S. Walker.

INDEX

acid rain 27
addiction 23-4
advertising 24-5
Africa 25,35
AIDS 24
air pollution 26
alcohol 23,38
allergies 8,29,32
alveoli 4,8-9,11,14,23,30,32,38,40
anaesthetics 38-9
    local 39
antibiotics 21,30,36
artificial ventilation 41
    iron lung 41
    ventilators 7,40
Asia 35
asthma 26-7,29,32-2
athletes 13,42
atmosphere 4

bacteria 21,34-5
bloodstream 4,8,16,39,40
blood vessels 10,14,17
bone marrow 42
brain 14,16
bronchioles 4,14,23,26-7,30
bronchitis 22,26,30
bronchus 4

cancer 22-3,26,30
capillaries 8-10
carbon dioxide 4,6,8-10,14,16,40,42,44
carbon monoxide 23,27
cells 8-10,21-2
chemicals 4,10,23,26-7,30
China 25
colds 18-19,21,30
cot deaths 16
cystic fibrosis 36-7

decongestants 21
diaphragm 5,7,13
DNA 21,36
dust mites 28-9

emphysema 22,30
energy 4,10,13
epiglottis 4
exercise 13

flu 18-19,21,30
France 24

gas masks 26
genes 36-7
    therapy 37
government 24

haemoglobin 8,23
hay fever 18,29
high altitude 42
hydrocarbons 27
hyperventilate 16
hysteria 16

immune system 21
India 25
intercostal muscle 21

Koch, Robert 34

larynx 4
Legionnaire's disease 30
lungs 4,6-8,10,13-14,16-17,22-3,26-7,34,42,43

mucus 18-19,21,23,30

nitrogen 9,27
nitrogen dioxide 9,27

nose, the 4,11,17-19,21

oesophagus 4
oxygen 4.6.8-14,30,39,42,44
    concentrators 11
    lack of 10
ozone 27

pharynx 4
photosynthesis 44
physiotherapy 36
pneumonia 30
polio 41
Portugal 24
premature babies 7,40

Queen Victoria 39

receptors 14,16
respiratory distress syndrome 7

sinuses 17-18
sinusitis 18
smog 26
smoking 4,22-5
South America 25
steroids 33
sulphur dioxide 9,26-7
surfactant 7

tobacco 23
    industry 24
trachea 4,12,21
transplants 36
tuberculosis (TB) 34-5

vehicle exhausts 4,26-7
viruses 19,21

X-ray 34

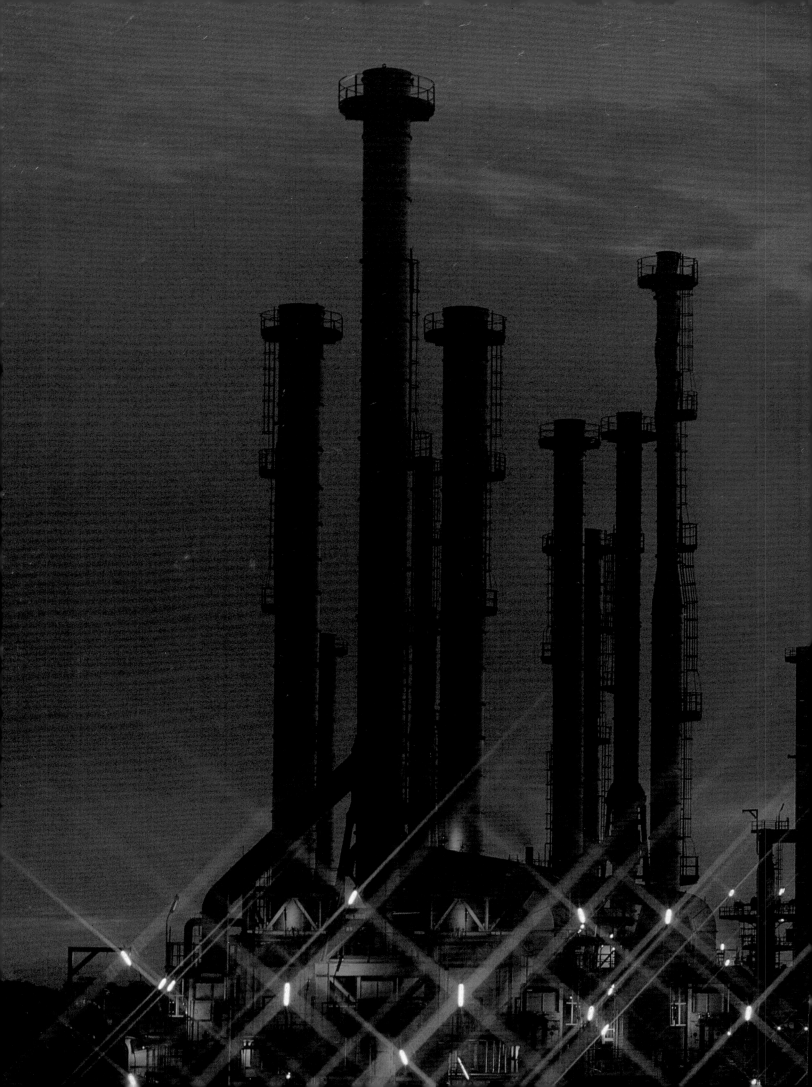

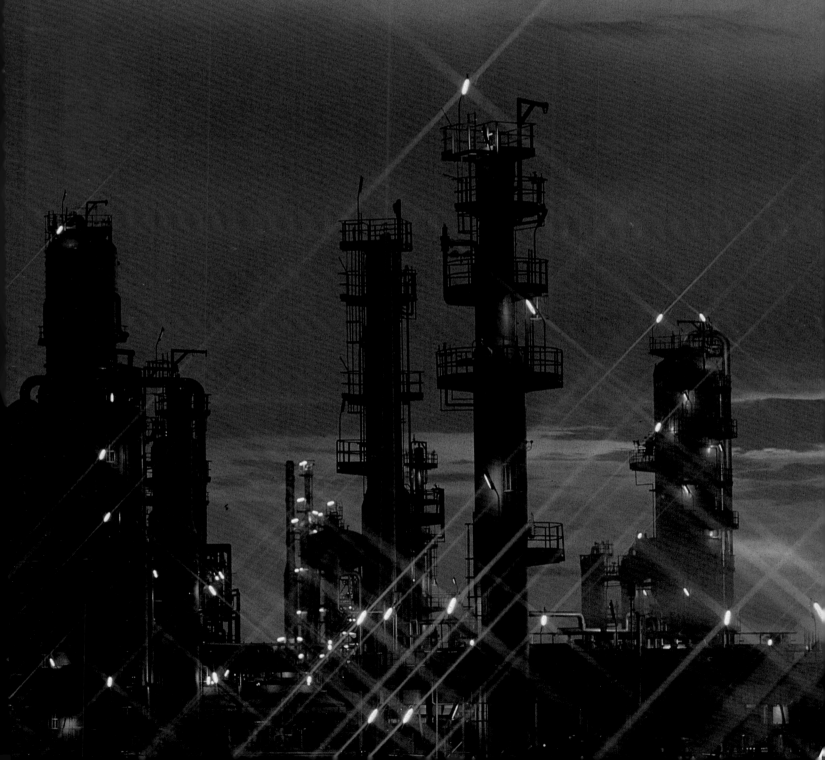

NIGERIA
A JUBILEE JOURNEY

ACKNOWLEDGEMENTS

The Publishers wish to record their appreciation for
the assistance and co-operation received from the
Federal Ministry of Information and Culture in
collecting materials for this book, the Federal Ministry
of Mines, Power and Steel and the Nigerian
Commission for National Museum of Arts and
Monuments for permission to take photographs of
artworks and artefacts from the various museums in
the country.

First published in 1988 by
Scorpion Publishing Ltd
Victoria House, Victoria Road
Buckhurst Hill, Essex IG9 5ES, England

ISBN 0 905906 78 0

Edited by Leonard Harrow and John Orley
Art direction and design: Colin Larkin
Studio assistant: Andrew Nash
Production assistants: Sue Pipe and Kay Larkin

All the photographs in this volume were specially
commissioned and taken by Jeff Jones,
Shell Photographic Services, London, except plates
107 and 108 which are courtesy of
All-Sport Photographic Limited
Photographic assistant: Andy Giddings

Typeset in Linotype New Baskerville 12 on 14 point
Printed on Parilux Matt 135gsm
Printed and bound in England by Jolly and Barber Ltd

CONTENTS

7   PREFACE

9   FOREWORD

11   THE LAND

31   WILDLIFE

37   PEOPLES OF NIGERIA

59   ART AND CULTURE

85   ARCHITECTURE

97   AGRICULTURE

105   TRADE, TRANSPORT AND INDUSTRY

121   ENERGY AND OIL

133   SPORT

137   EDUCATION AND HEALTH

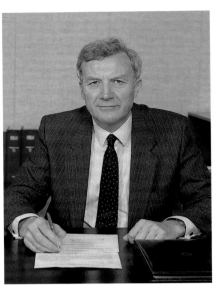

Mr Brian Lavers, Chairman and Managing Director of Shell Nigeria

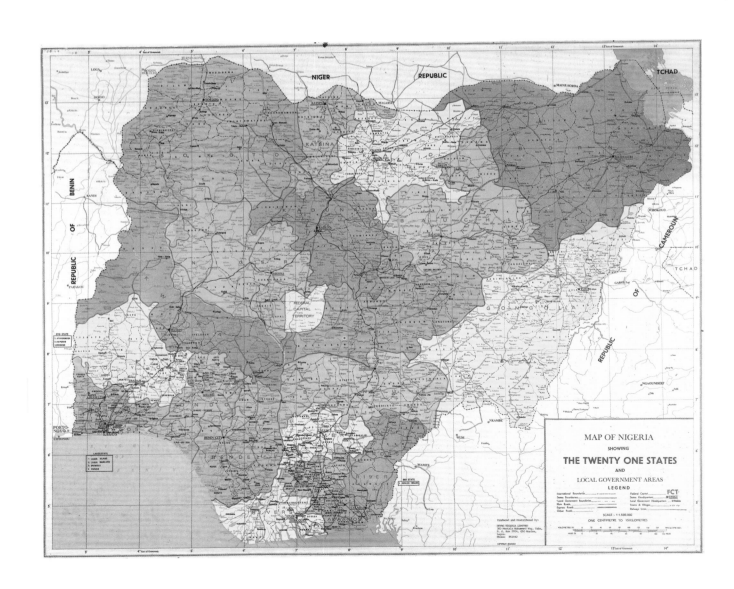

MAP OF NIGERIA

SHOWING

THE TWENTY ONE STATES

AND

LOCAL GOVERNMENT AREAS

PREFACE

1988 is the Golden Jubilee year of Shell's partnership with Nigeria in the exploration and development of her oil and gas resources, a most fruitful venture, bringing wealth and prosperity to a great nation. We are pleased to invite you to celebrate with us.

Although the first petroleum exploration took place in Nigeria as early as 1908, systematic scientific surveys of the country really began with the arrival of Shell in 1938. Even then, success came very slowly. The key to unravelling the complex petroleum geology of Nigeria was not easy to find, particularly with the relatively simple exploration techniques available to us in the early years. The first commercial oil discovery was made in 1956 at Oloibiri, after eighteen long years of patient work in the difficult terrain of swamps and estuaries.

Because of the significance of this discovery to the economy, development began at once and only two years later Nigeria had joined the ranks of petroleum exporting countries. There then followed a whole series of exploration successes which formed the foundations of to-day's great industry. A huge infra-structure of facilities was developed to handle a peak production of 1.5 million barrels per day, including 83 producing oil fields with over 1,000 wells, 1,700 kilometres of pipelines, innumerable processing plants and two major export terminals with offshore loading buoys to receive the world's largest tankers.

From 1962 onwards, other oil companies joined in the search for hydrocarbons. But, even to-day Shell, as operator for the NNPC/Shell joint venture, is proud to be producing over half of Nigeria's oil and gas, which itself contributes 95 per cent of the nation's foreign exchange earnings. Far from resting on its laurels, Shell in its jubilee year is planning to invest more than ever before in the continued growth of the industry. Between January and August, 1988, Shell announced five new oil and gas discoveries amounting to 160 million barrels of oil and and 250 billion cubic feet of gas.

The future of the industry will be based not only on oil but also on gas. In its 50th year Shell with NNPC has completed a major project at Utorogu to supply gas to Lagos. Moreover as Technical Leader of the NNPC/Shell/Agip/Elf Nigeria LNG project it will be instrumental in exporting liquified natural gas to the world and initiating a new and major source of export earnings for Nigeria in the 1990s and beyond.

In offering this book, *Nigeria – A Jubilee Journey*, we are paying homage to the great nation we serve. It is first and foremost a pictorial essay, recording the beauty of the land, the wild life and the people, the arts and crafts, the architecture and costumes that together express Nigeria's history, the industry, agriculture and educational system that have built modern Nigeria, and finally the nation at play, dancing, singing and riding at traditional ceremonies and exciting us all with the excellence of her Olympic sportsmen and sportswomen.

No Jubilee Journey would be complete without some descriptive text to stimulate the imagination of the traveller. We have therefore included a short history of the country that goes back so many times further than the modest fifty years that are encompassed by Shell's own contribution. We have also traced some background to the things we see, especially the craftwork and many beautiful artefacts. It is impossible in a handful of photographs and a short textual sketch to capture the whole essence of Nigeria. Our only hope is that these small random vignettes will give an impression, however inadequate, of the country and of its people.

Brian Lavers

BRIAN A. LAVERS
MANAGING DIRECTOR, SHELL PETROLEUM
DEVELOPMENT CO. OF NIGERIA LTD.

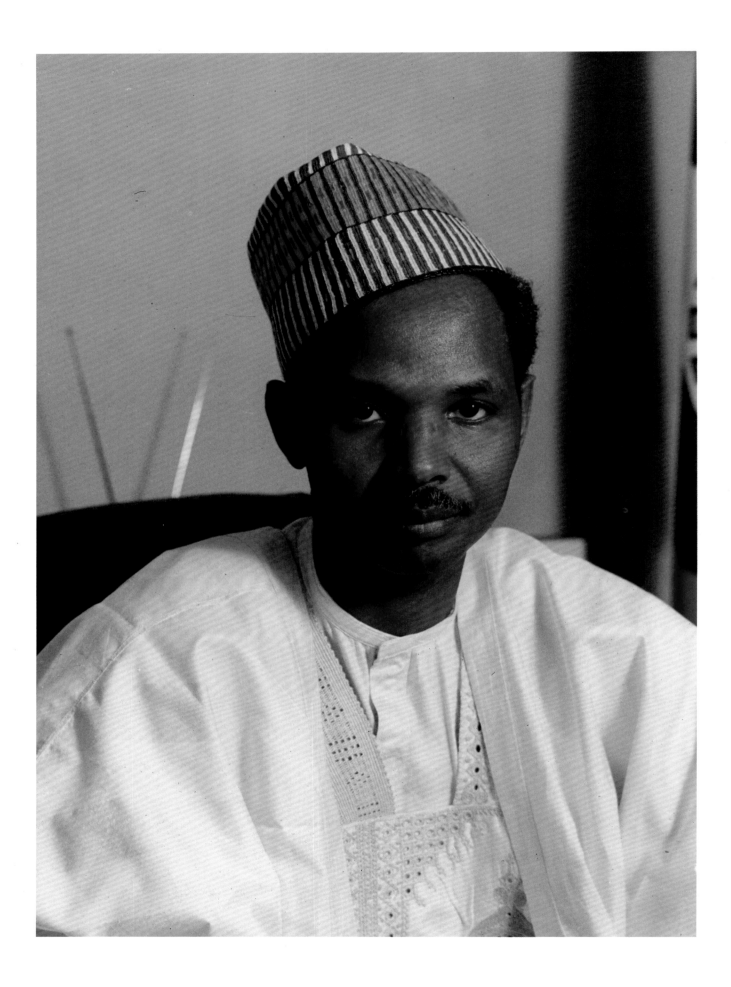

FOREWORD

BY ALHAJI RILWANU LUKMAN
THE HONOURABLE MINISTER OF
PETROLEUM RESOURCES
FEDERAL REPUBLIC OF NIGERIA

I am delighted to have been invited to write a short foreword to this book published by The Shell Development Company of Nigeria Limited to commemorate its Golden Jubilee Anniversary.

The last half century has witnessed amazing changes and steadfast progress in Nigeria as vividly portrayed in the various sections of this book. The progress shown points to a future of great promise and the significant role that the oil industry has played and will continue to play in the economic and social development of the nation.

The beautiful illustrations portray distinguishing characteristics of the diverse landscape, culture, traditions, agricultural and industrial development of Nigeria.

In giving us such a gift on its birthday, Shell is not only restating its importance in Nigeria's energy industry but is also demonstrating its long term commitment to the society and environment of our beloved country.

Perhaps we should even now look forward to the next milestone in Nigeria and Shell's story and hope that it will also be celebrated in such a worthy and handsome manner.

It is my great pleasure to introduce this book to a wider public in Nigeria and around the world and so help to promote greater understanding of Nigeria amongst our friends old and new.

RILWANU LUKMAN

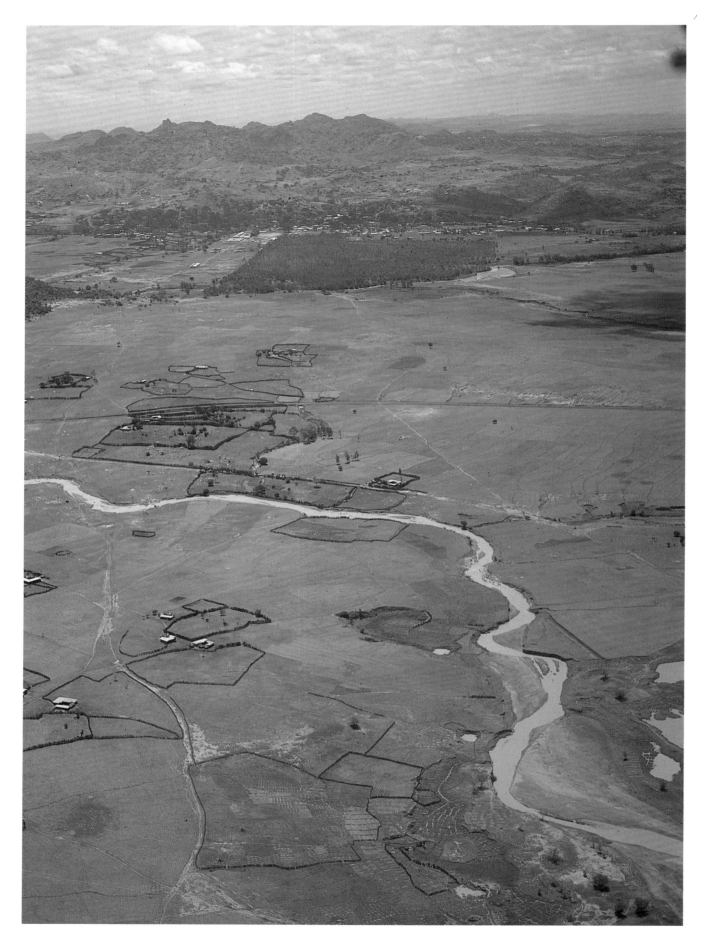

Jos Plateau, Plateau State

THE LAND

NIGERIA is situated in West Africa on the Gulf of Guinea and bounded by the countries of Cameroon in the south east, Chad to the north east, Niger to the north and Benin to the west. These boundaries are a relatively recent creation. In spite of hills, rivers and plateau areas no major natural boundaries exist, apart from the Atlantic Ocean to the south. However, the terrain is often difficult, with forests and swamps in the southern zone, and thus rivers and their tributaries form the natural arteries of communication.

Nigeria is at present the most populous nation in Africa and has long been one of the most prominent in terms of culture and civilisation. At various times in its history it has been the site of civilisations counted amongst the most powerful and prosperous of the continent with a consequent flowering of art and sophisticated workmanship in many fields.

Nigeria is a federal republic. Having once been part of the British colonial presence in Africa it now participates as an independent and very important partner in the organisation of the Commonwealth. The present capital is Lagos but a new Federal capital is being constructed at Abuja which is more centrally placed within the country. With a population in 1981 of over 79 million and present estimate of over 100 million and a land area of 923,773 square kilometres, Nigeria ranks as one of the most important nations in the world.

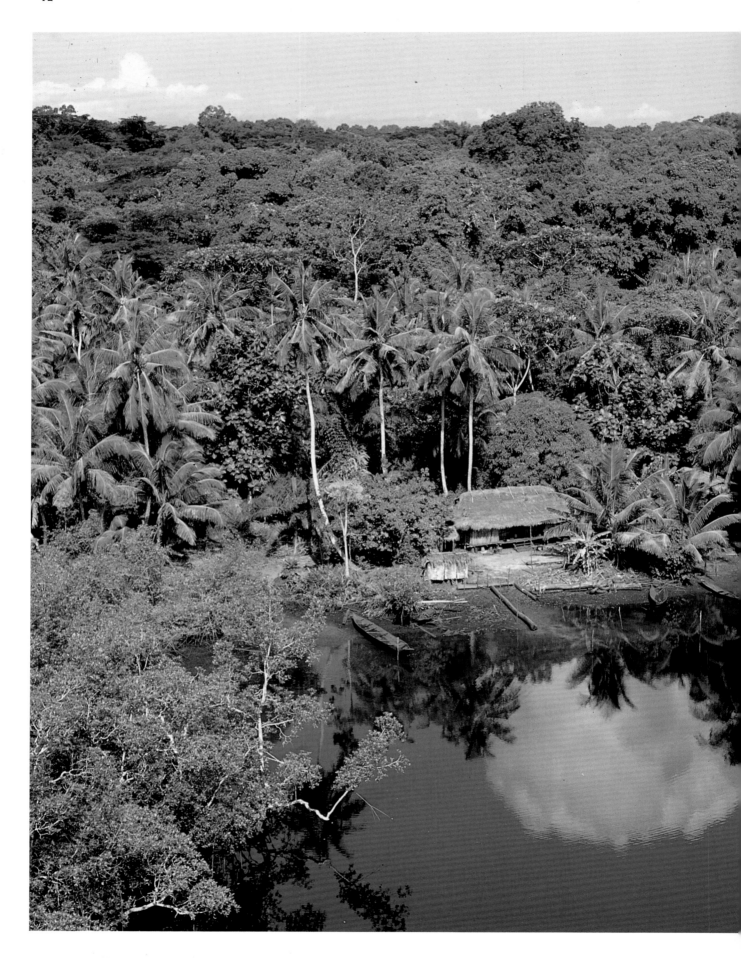

Village in Bendel State

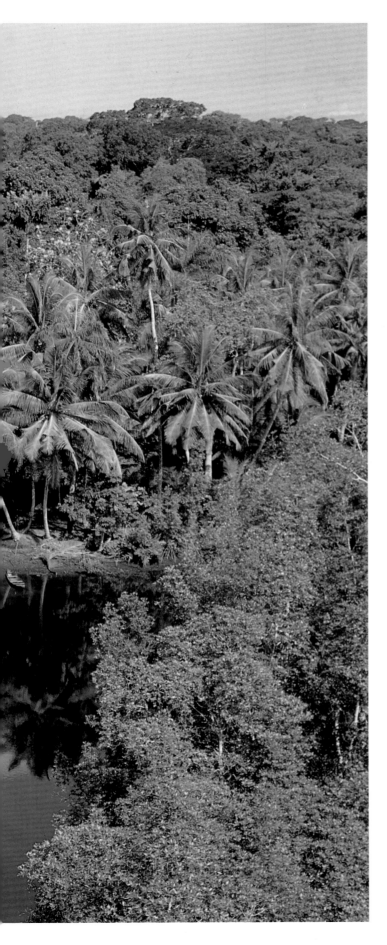

THE NIGER AND THE BENUE

The key natural feature of the area is the river from which Nigeria takes its name. Its confluence with the Benue provides a natural focus for the whole country before flowing into the many distributaries which go to form the Niger Delta. These rivers have throughout the ages enabled an exchange and cross fertilization of cultures and have united the peoples in the area. In this sense Nigeria is a common entity, despite its diversity in cultural manifestations.

The River Niger has always been the most important communications artery, as well as a means of sustenance, providing irrigation for the dry savannah, and fish for those who live along its banks.

The river rises in the Futa Jallon highlands in present-day Guinea and runs north-east into Mali, then turns south-east to Bussa before it is joined by the Benue at Lokoja.

As the most significant means of communication and sustenance it naturally developed important market towns along its banks, as at Lokoja, Aboh, Onitsha and Asaba. The delta towns of Brass and Bonny also became important markets.

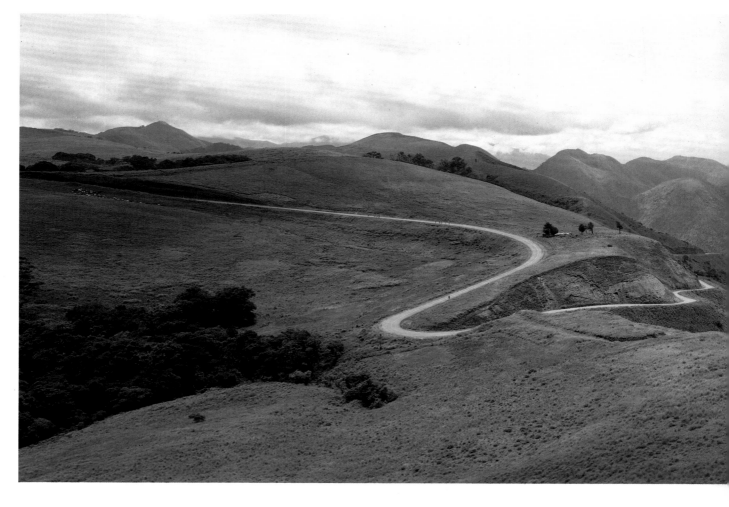

Obudu cattle ranch, Cross River State

THE ORIGIN OF NIGER AND NIGERIA

The origin of the word 'Niger' is obscure. Some theorise that it is derived from the Latin word meaning 'black'; others, that *Nijer*, or *Njer*, is a name of African origin conferred on the river by a local community; there also exists the possibility that 'Niger' is derived from the Greek *naghar* meaning 'river'. Although the influence of Latin and Greek colonies in North Africa during early history and the Classical leanings of European colonists at a later stage may have some bearing on this, it is more than likely that the name was indeed conferred by African communities.

The word 'Nigeria' to describe the whole area surrounding the river was first used in 1897 by Flora Shaw, a correspondent for *The Times*, to describe the Royal Niger Company's territories. Her husband was Brigadier-General Frederick Lugard, who in 1900, following his wife's example, named the territories of the Royal Niger Company 'Northern Nigeria'. The whole country became known as Nigeria in 1914 when Northern Nigeria and Southern Nigeria were amalgamated into one entity under the governorship of Lugard.

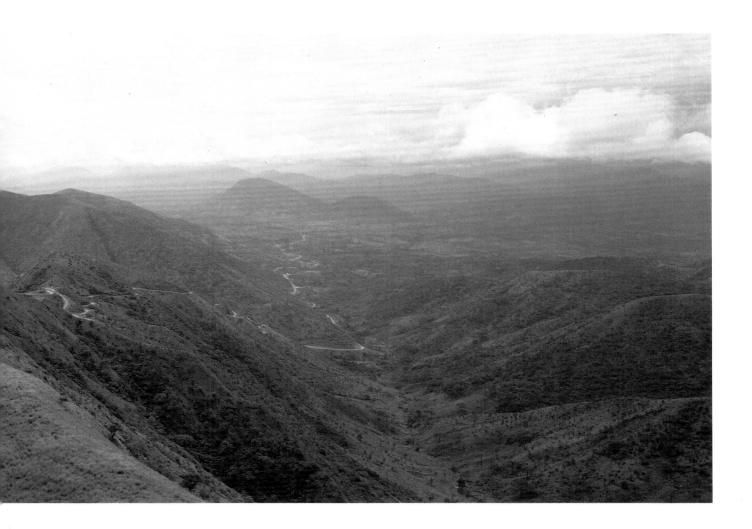

GEOGRAPHIC ZONES

The natural geographic zones of the country
have greatly influenced the development of
culture and political structures amongst
Nigerian peoples. The zones fall into several
distinct categories. In the south along the
coast the climate is marked by heavy rainfall
and the vegetation consists chiefly of
saltwater mangrove swamps. Next to this
zone is the region of thick forest, again
characterised by heavy rainfall. Further north
where the rainfall decreases is the semi-
savannah, and in the far north of the country
lies true savannah – vast areas of open
grassland with very little rainfall. Directly to
the north of the savannah region lies the
Sahara Desert.

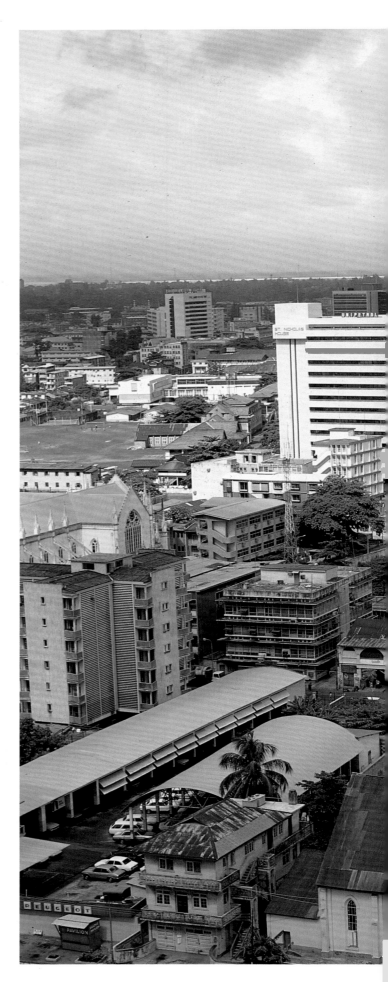

Old and new buildings, Lagos

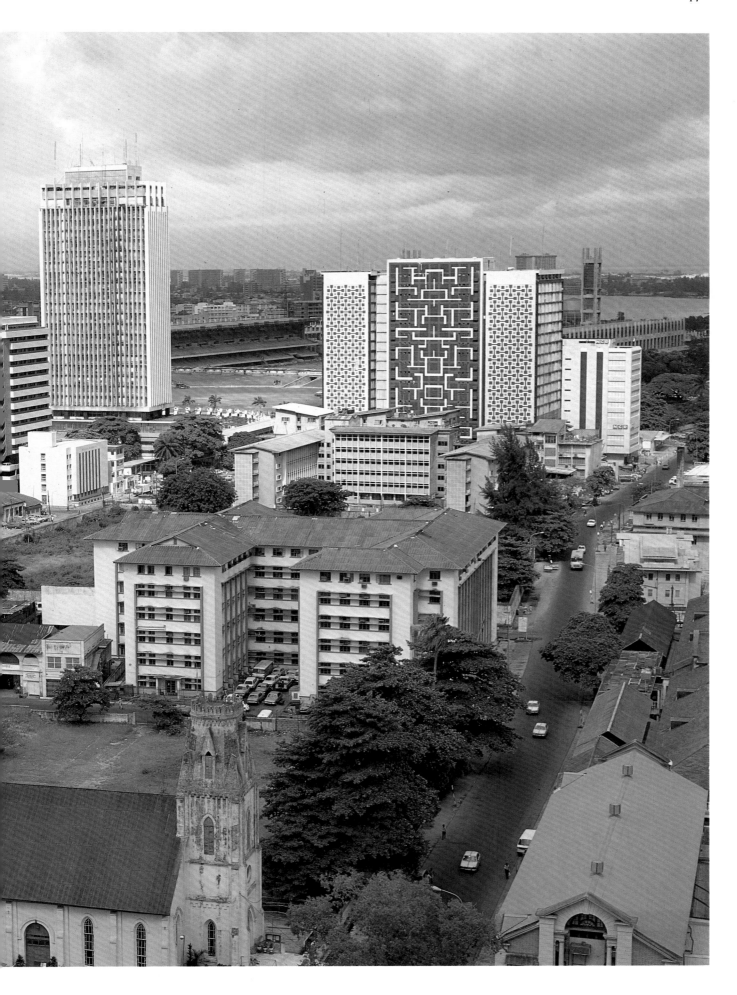

**Fishing on the River Niger with Murtala Mohammed Bridge, Lokoja,
Kwara State, in the background**

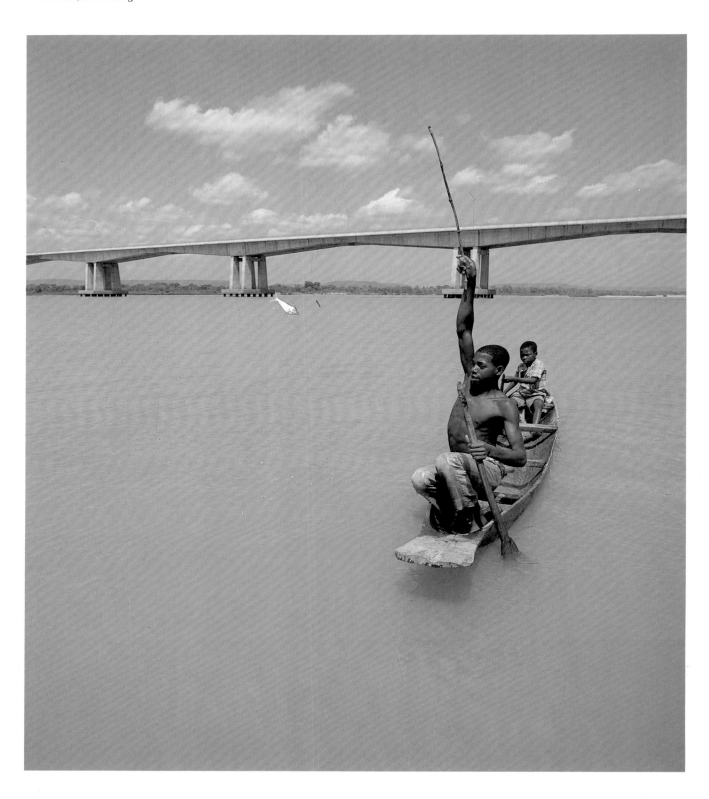

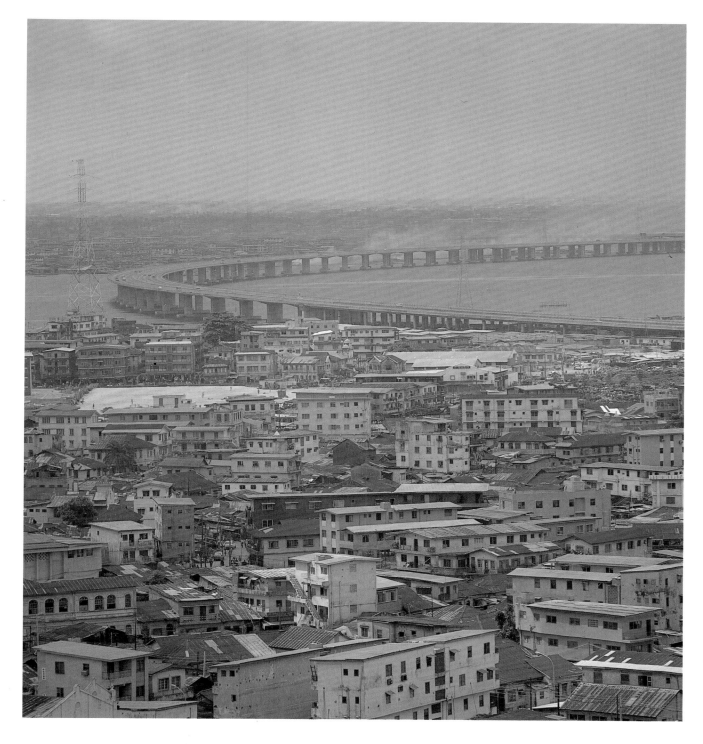

Lagos, looking towards Victoria Island

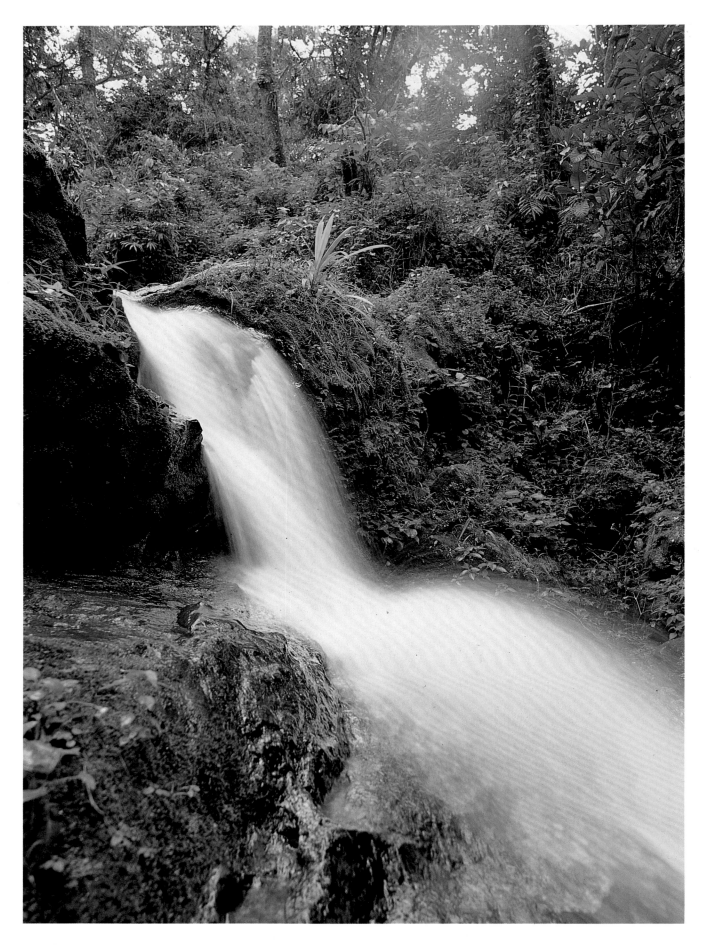

Waterfall in Obudu cattle ranch, Cross River State

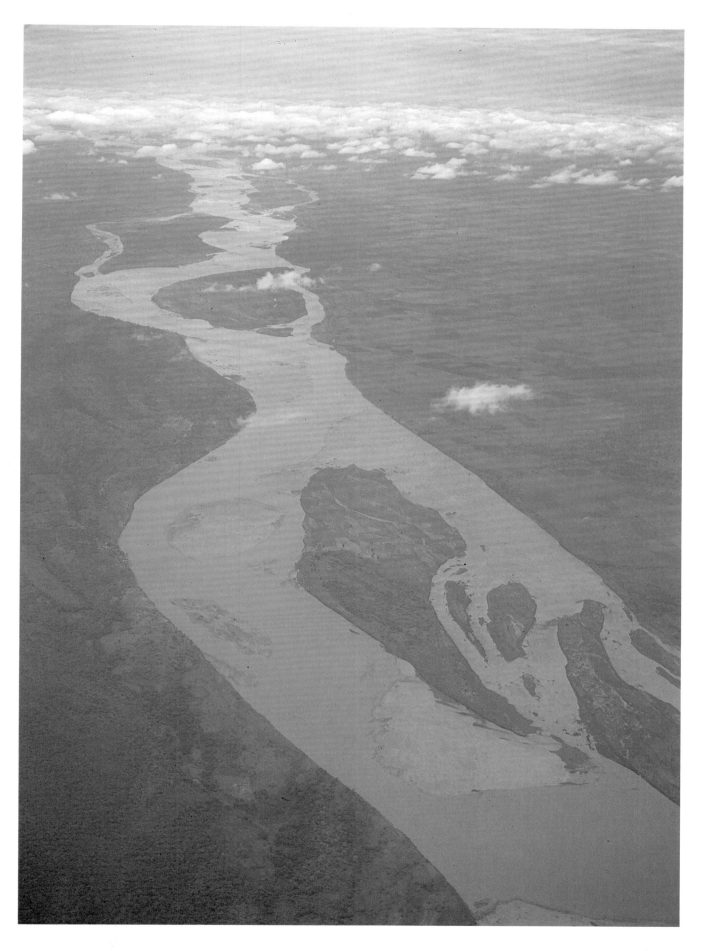

The River Benue on its course through Benue State

Old Finima village, near Port Harcourt

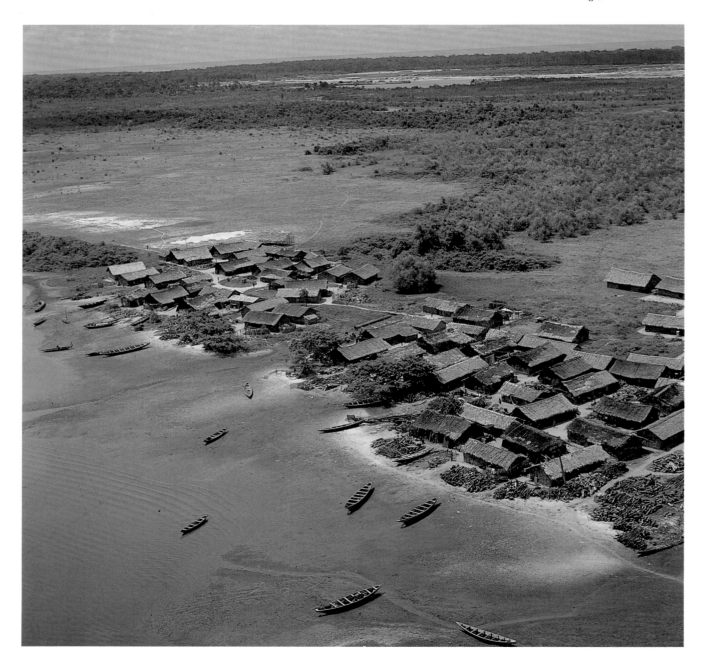

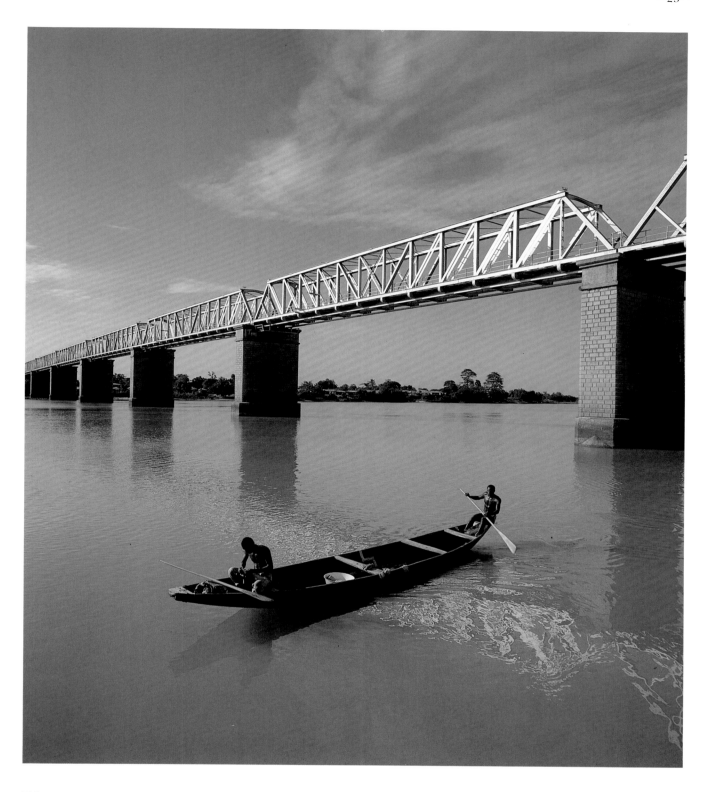

Fishermen on the River Niger passing by Old Jebba Bridge, Niger State

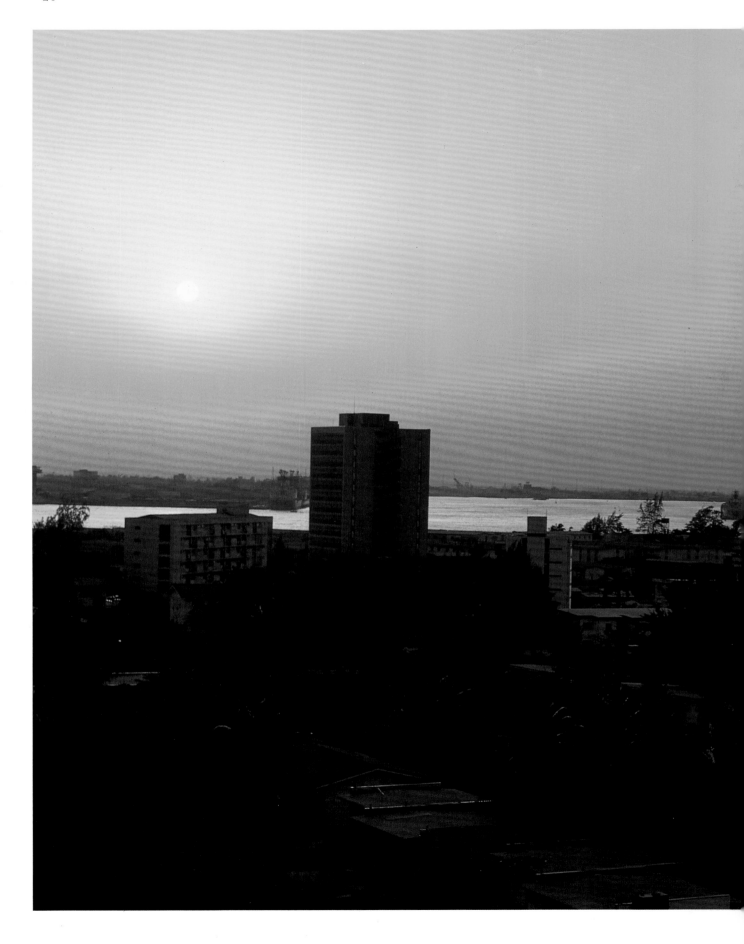

Lagos Island at sunset

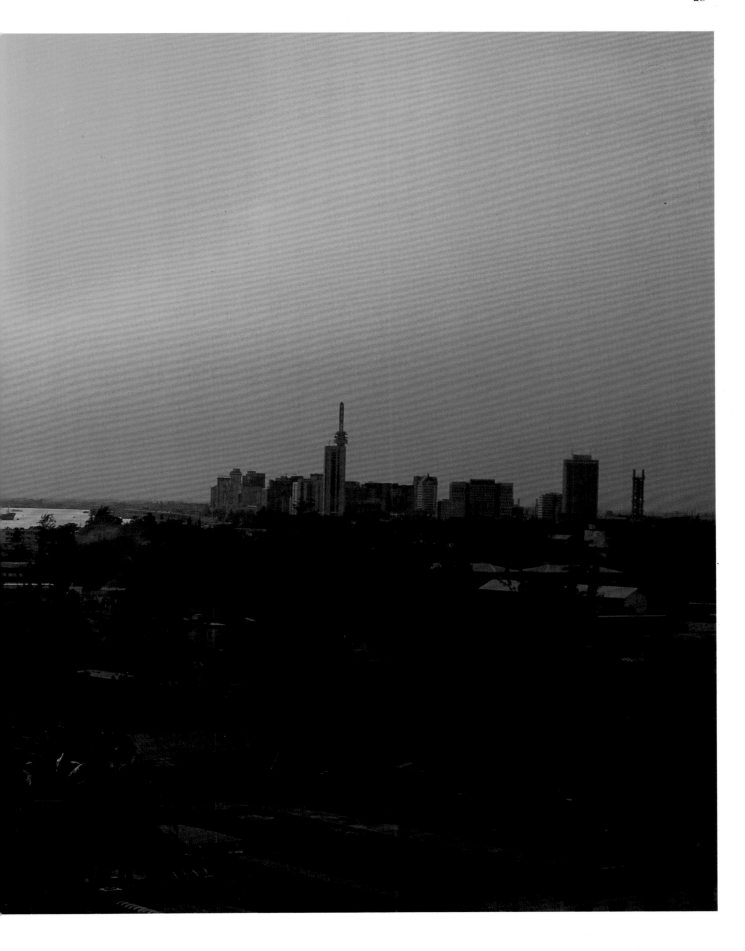

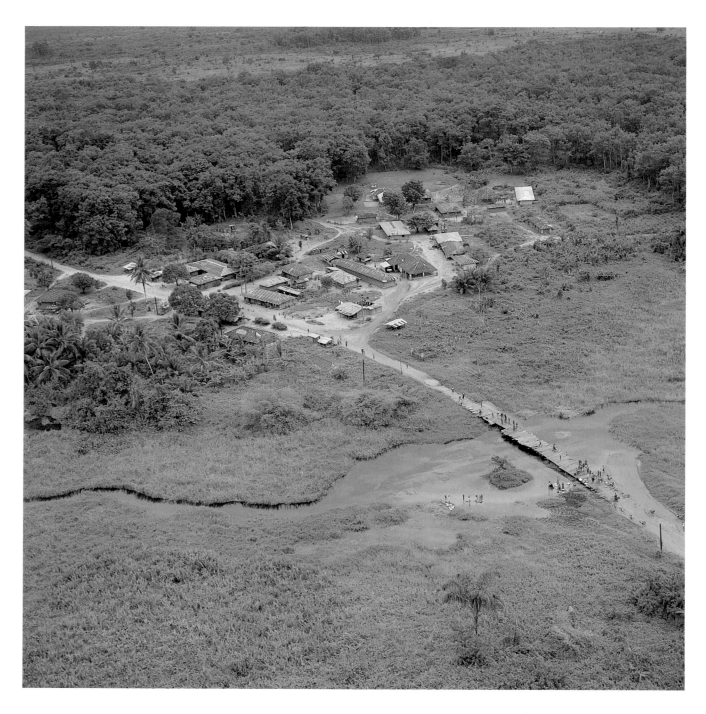

Abraka 1 village, Bendel State

Badagry Beach in Lagos State

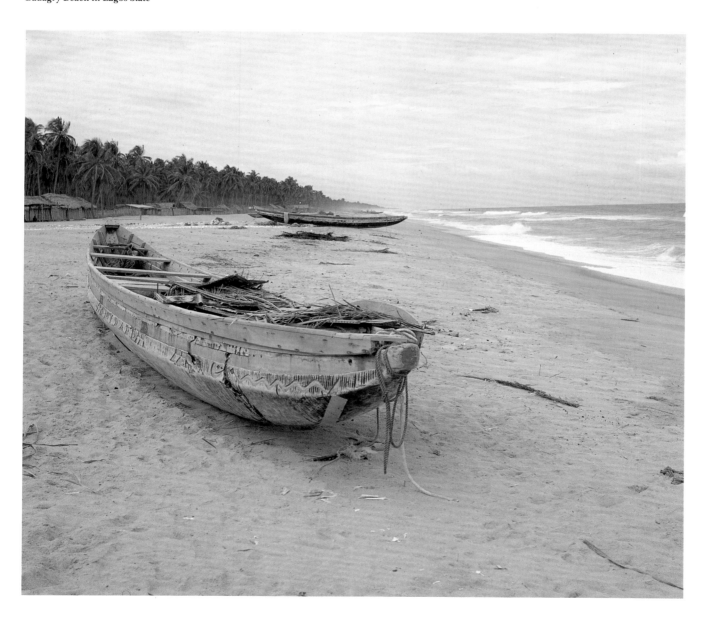

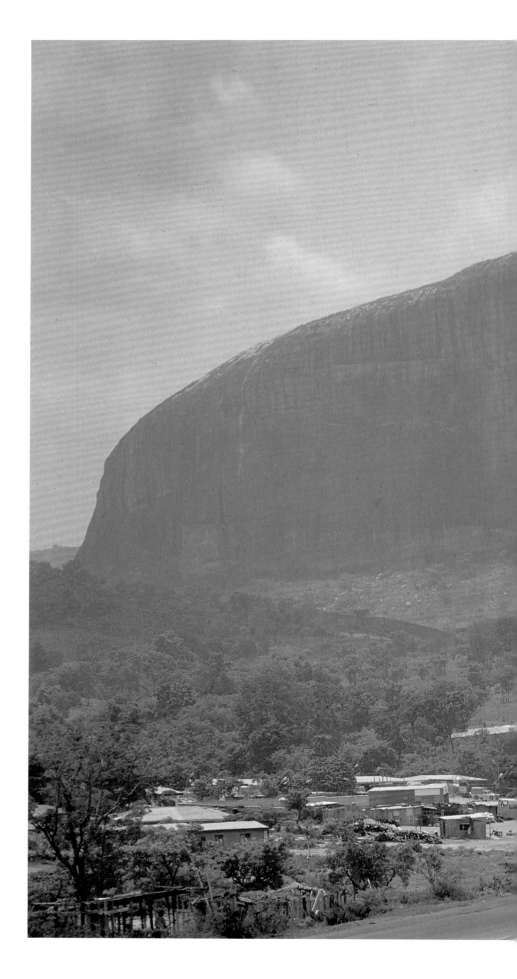

Zuma Rock, Abuja, Federal Capital Territory

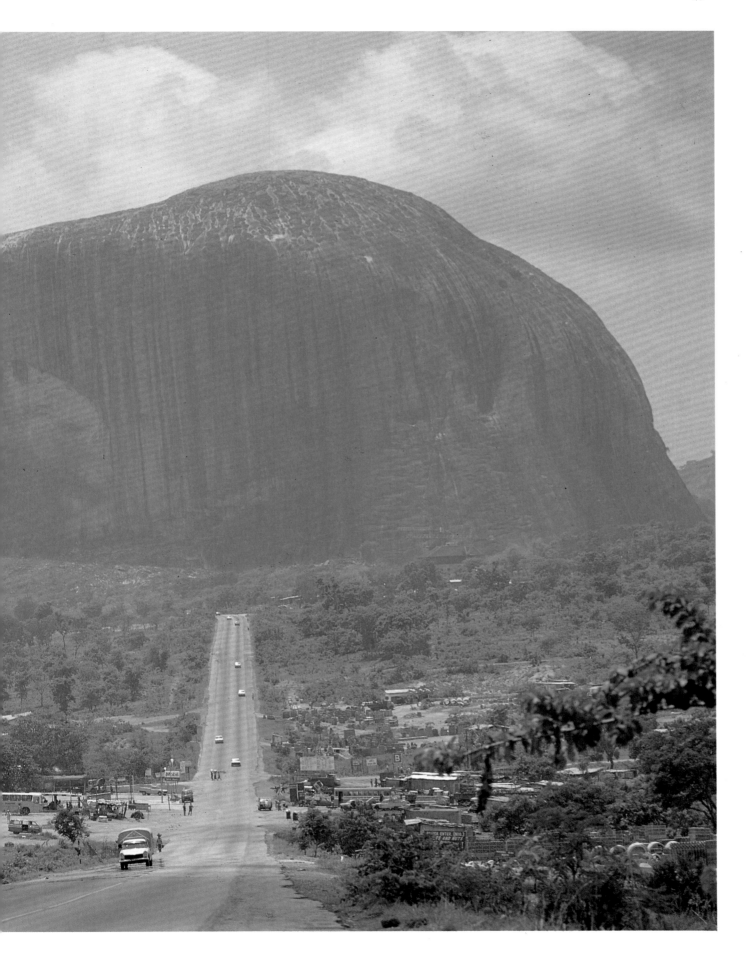

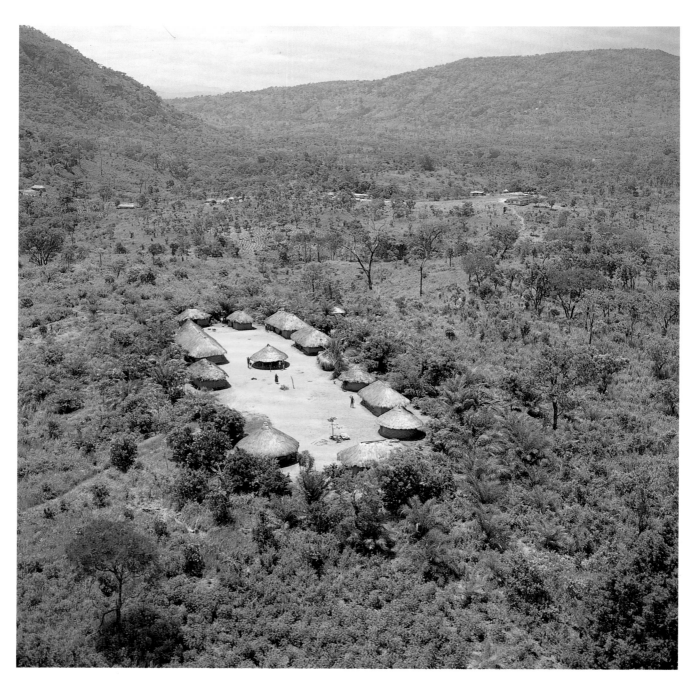

Village near Obudu, Cross River State

WILDLIFE

NIGERIA is rich in flora and fauna. The three distinct geographical zones to a large extent dictate their distribution, although several species have managed to adapt themselves to widely contrasting habitats.

The mangrove swamps, lagoons and creeks of southern Nigeria naturally abound in amphibious vertebrates such as frogs, river turtles, crocodiles and hippopotamus. Birds are generally of the wader type since they depend on water creatures for their nourishment. Their long legs for paddling at the edge of waves and long bills for probing the sand or mud are ideally suited for this purpose.

Tree and ground dwelling animals inhabit the middle rainforest belt. Among the larger varieties are monkeys, chimpanzees, leopards and elephants. Other smaller mammals include rodents and fruitbats. Insects are numerous in this environment, as are reptiles, especially lizards and a large variety of snakes. Birdlife is especially rich, including such species as parrots and guinea fowl.

The savannah area of Nigeria abounds in grass eaters, runners and hoppers. Large herbivores, mainly ungulates such as horses, camels and gazelles, and small rodents exist in great numbers and varieties. There are also hyenas, lions and leopards and other carnivores. The area is rich in invertebrates and insect life. Among the birds, seed and insect eaters predominate in this type of environment. With local populations rearing large herds of cattle and grass-grazing animals existing in great numbers the cattle egret is a common sight. The common vulture and ostrich are also to be seen.

For the ornithologist, Nigeria has an extensive variety of birds. There is also an almost inexhaustible area in the forests and bush for the entomologists in search of butterflies, moths, beetles and other forms of insect.

A number of game reserves have been established in Nigeria where animals can multiply and flourish. The Yankari Game Reserve with its warm springs and the Borgu Game Reserve near Kainji offer opportunities for visitors to see some rare species of Nigerian wildlife in their natural habitat. Wildlife species in the Yankari Reserve include elephant, lion, cheetah, hartebeest, hippopotamus, monkeys, reptiles and a wide range of birds.

The University of Ibadan has a zoo with a sizeable number of examples of Nigerian wildlife. The Anambra State government also maintains a zoo in Enugu while there are others in Jos, Kano and Ikogosi.

The Nigerian Conservation Foundation (NCF), in affiliation with the World Wildlife Fund (recently renamed the Worldwide Fund for Nature), has been engaged in various important projects in Nigeria aimed at saving the best natural areas from further damage. Some of the most interesting work undertaken by the NCF includes the protection of certain endemic primate species

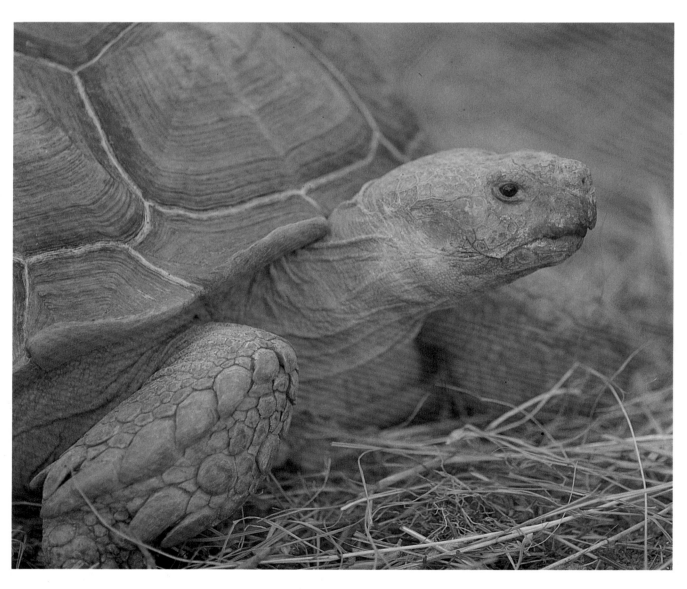

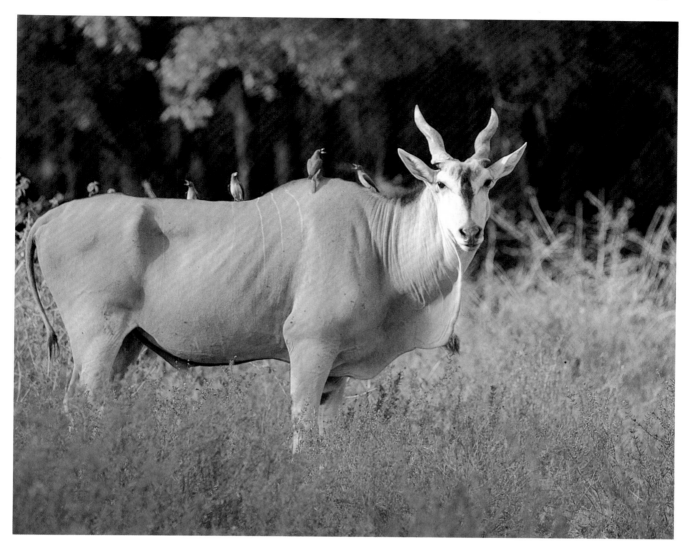

opposite: A tortoise in Bauchi State

above: A female eland with hornbill companions

in the Okomu Forest Reserve in Bendel State; other mammals, birds and reptiles have also been included in this sanctuary. Another significant conservation programme undertaken by the NCF is in the Cross River State for the protection of the moist tropical forest which supports a viable population of lowland gorillas (white-nosed Guenon and Mona). The uniqueness and beauty of this undisturbed rain forest with its enormous variety of both flora and fauna has a unique beauty.

Some of the rarest monkeys in the world have also been located in the Oguta area on the border of Imo State and Rivers State and are in need of protection. In view of the alarming rate at which the natural habitat is being destroyed on the Lekki Peninsula, conservation work here has been given high priority. Other plans involve the preservation of the important relic high forest area on the Jos Plateau and management plans for the Yankari Game Reserve in Bauchi State and the Gashaka-Gunti Game Reserve in Gongola State. The value of the environment and the commitment to its protection is fully endorsed by the major industries of Nigeria, especially the oil industry.

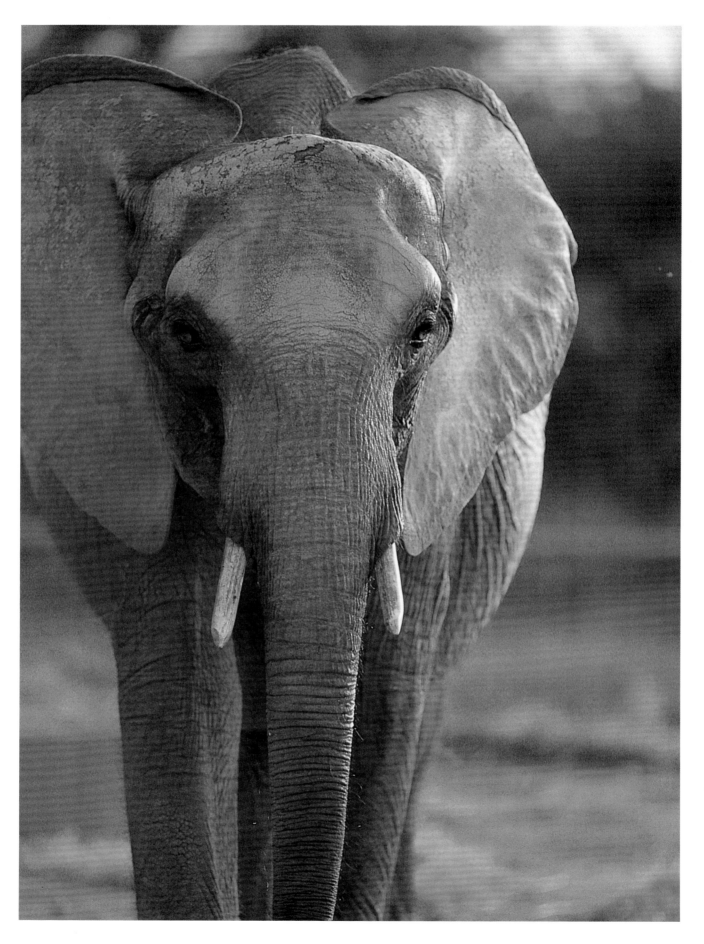

African savannah elephant

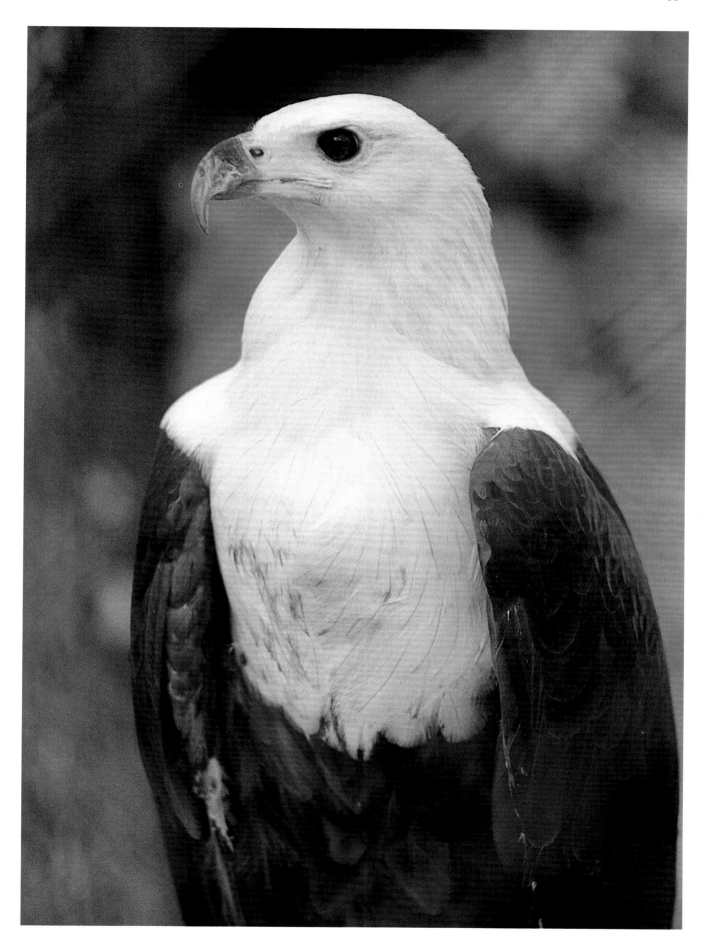

African river eagle, photographed in Bauchi State

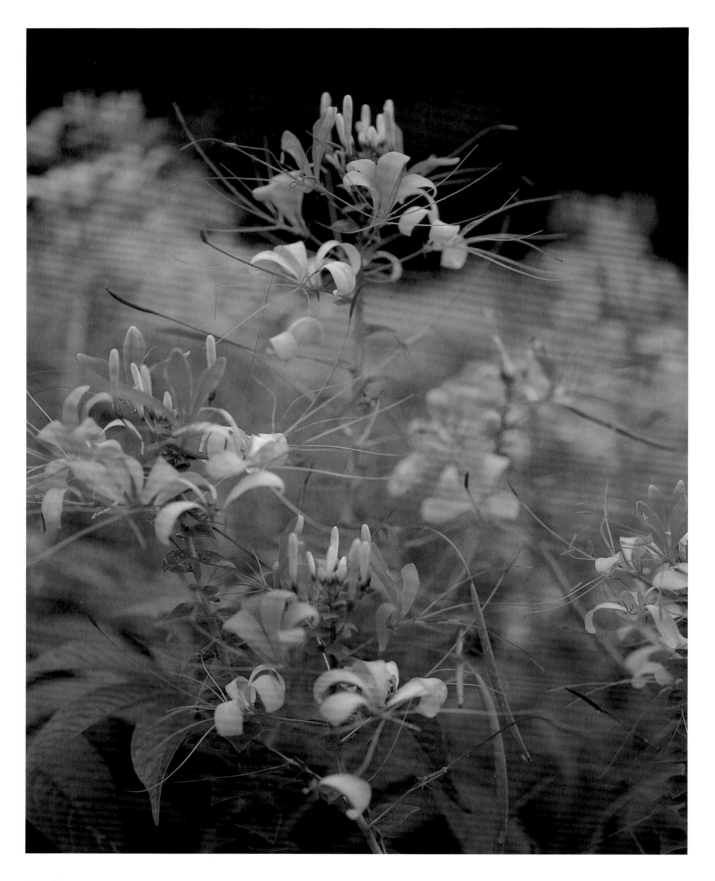

Tiger lilies

PEOPLES OF NIGERIA

THE diversity of local culture within Nigeria manifests itself in the diversity of ethnic and language groups. In the past language groups have often formed political units, such as the Hausa states, the Edo people of the Benin Empire, the Jukun, the Igbo and the Yoruba. The Hausa, amongst whom the Fulani, Kanuri, Kano and Katsina are prominent, occupy the northern savannah zone. Peoples such as the Jukun inhabited the middle zone along the Niger, as did other peoples such as the Egbira, Idoma, Igbo, Tiv and Yoruba. The Aro occupy the east of Igboland and the Efik and Ijaw the far south along the Niger Delta. Other peoples include the Angas, Biron, Edo, Ibibio, Igala, Isoko, Itshekiri, Kanem, Nupe and Urhobo. At present there are three predominant tribal groupings, the Hausa/Fulani, the Yoruba and the Igbo, who occupy approximately the north, west and east of the country respectively.

DEVELOPMENT OF CULTURES

In the swampy coastal areas of the south, where no agriculture was possible because of the salt water and mangroves, the people developed an economy based on fishing and salt making, which products they exchanged for crops and food produced further inland. Consequently much of their skills and cultural traditions involved the use of canoes and river transportation, whereas the rather different environment of the neighbouring forest areas produced peoples dependent on hunting skills. Since it was here that Europeans first penetrated the country the dominant religion has been Christianity, although, as elsewhere, there is a considerable number of traditional animists as well as some Muslims.

By contrast, the savannah in the north enabled the development of an economy based on livestock and herding, notably of horses and cattle. In particular, peoples of the north were famed for their prowess as riders and the festivals which displayed those skills. With the grassland and the Sahara Desert constituting a difficult but less impenetrable barrier than the dense forests to the south the area came under the dominant influence of the Islamic religion and its civilisation. In fact, for long periods of history the northern peoples were members of states which stretched well beyond the present borders of northern Nigeria. Despite the differences, the interdependence of peoples and the cultural parallels between them are quite striking. There are great similarities, for example, in creation and flood myths and common details within a wide variety of festivals and cultural rites.

EARLIEST OCCUPATION

The earliest occupation of Nigeria has been traced by archaeologists as far back as 65,000 BC. Material evidence of human existence has been provided by a skeleton found at Iwo Eleru near Akure in Ondo State dated around 10,000 BC. Artefacts have been found within the country from each of the three main Stone Age periods.

The Early Stone Age can be dated from around 3,000,000 to 35,000 BC. Evidence of this occupation has been provided by tools of the Oldowan type (named after Olduvai Gorge in Tanzania), which consist of bone, wood and stone for chopping and cutting. The Middle Stone Age, from approximately 35,000 to 12,000 BC, provided Acheulian type tools (after St Acheul in northern France). These tools were made in the Early Stone Age and continued to be perfected in the Middle Stone Age. They consisted of hand axes, of oval shapes, trimmed on both sides to provide cutting edges. Such tools have been discovered on Jos Plateau. Other tools include small stone hunting tools which have been found also at Afikpo in Imo State, Jos Plateau, Iwo Eleru in Ondo State and Mejiro cave in Old Oyo. Sangoan tools, which were efficient choppers somewhat like picks and so called because they were first discovered at Sango Bay on the shores of Lake Victoria, Uganda, have also been found in Nigeria in the upper Sokoto River, Sokoto State.

The Late Stone Age in Nigeria may be considered to range from roughly 12,000 to 500 BC, by the end of which period some areas had already evolved Bronze and Early Iron Age cultures. It was characterized by the development of agriculture, including rice growing and efficient food storage techniques.

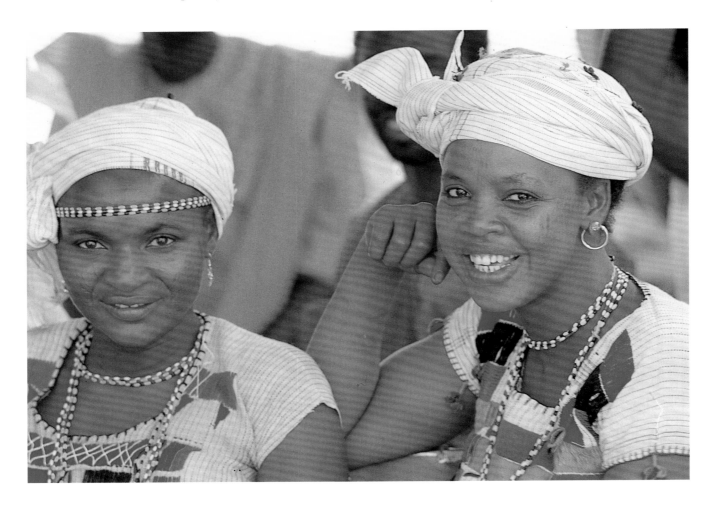

CULTURES UP TO THE 19TH CENTURY

The earlier phases of Nigeria's history are most admirably reflected in the series of important civilisations, which have left to posterity many exquisite works. These civilisations might be briefly considered in chronological order.

The Nok culture, so called as its earliest artefacts were found in the Nok area near the Niger-Benue confluence, is probably the earliest in the sub-Saharan region which practised iron smelting. Its main period was during the first millennium BC. The advantage given by this knowledge allowed the culture to become dominant over quite a large area and the savannah lands which the Nok inhabited became an agriculturally prosperous region.

opposite: Two young women attending the Katsina Sallah

below: Children in Lapai, Niger State

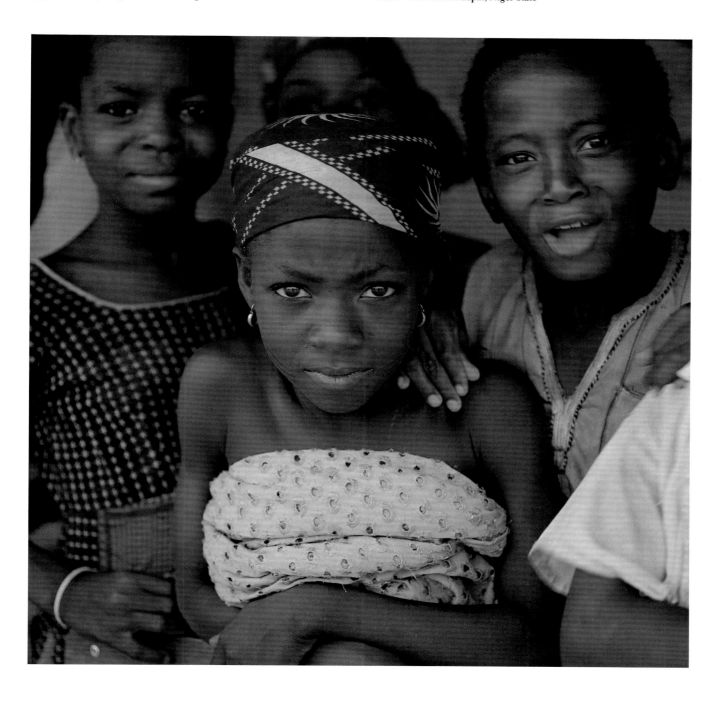

Surviving artefacts are characterised by a number of small terracotta sculptures of animals, and especially human heads. Their distinctive features are carefully drawn hairstyles and jewellery, usually hairbands and necklaces. The eyes of the figures are formed by a triangle with a hole for the pupil. Ears and hairlines were also often pierced suggesting that the sculptures were also originally adorned with other decorative features. Many of the heads have broken away from their original bodies. The original height of the complete sculptures is thought to have been about 1.2 metres. The technological skills of the Nok people and the wealth this gave them would explain the blossoming of the civilisation's artistry.

The sculptural traditions of Nigeria are continued in the remarkable artefacts created by the culture of Igbo-Ukwu in the 9th-10 centuries around Enugu, including bronze and copper objects with elaborate and complex surface decoration. Perhaps the greatest of such objects is the famous rope pot in the National Museum, Lagos. Made by the *cire perdue* method, the pot was cast in several sections as was the knotted rope which covers its surface which was itself bent to fit the object. The Igbo-Ukwu site was probably an ancient shrine or treasury. Apart from the great expertise shown by the artists, the sophistication of the society is further indicated by the fact that copper was not available locally and was probably brought across the Sahara from North Africa. Hence, Nigeria was involved at an early stage in extensive and far-flung trade.

The art of Ife, at its peak from the 12th to 15th centuries, shows the continued sophistication and wealth of Nigerian society.

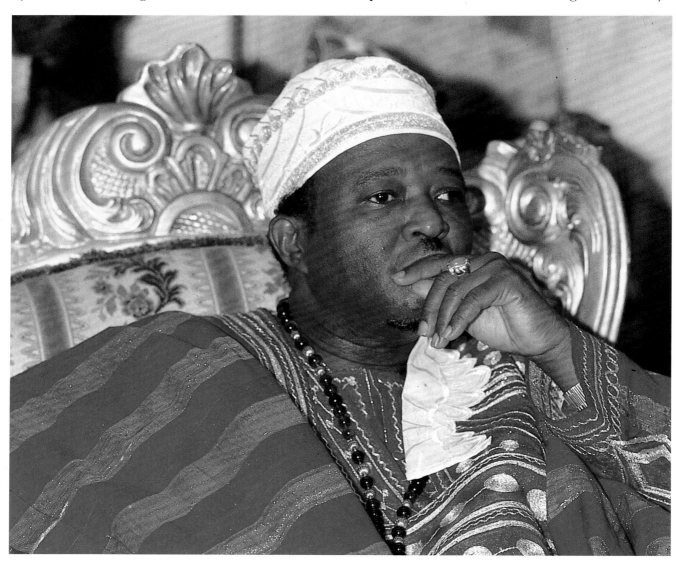

Ooni of Ife at his palace at Ile-Ife, Oyo State

Its art has come to us as a series of magnificent and stately figures and heads. Extremely lifelike, the bronze busts are believed to be of the kings, or *oonis*, of the region. The realism is emphasised by the scarification, the precise modelling and the elaborate headdresses. It is currently thought that these figures were supported on wooden bodies and formed part of elaborate burial rituals for the *ooni*. Within Yoruba tradition Ife is an important cult centre which grew wealthy on the tribute and offerings made by surrounding rulers thus enabling Ife to import copper from afar. Much influenced by Ife, and indeed Benin, is the art of Owo of the 15th century.

Traditionally Owo is said to have been founded by emigrants from Ife, and in its terracotta sculptures shows many features seen at Ife, such as the modelling of the eyes, the headdresses and scarification. The fame of Benin and its bronzes extends throughout the world. Between the 15th and 19th centuries, the *obas* of Benin were served by an exclusive group of craftsmen who produced magnificent artefacts for the court not only in bronze, but also in ivory and terracotta. Originally the metalworking tradition was influenced by Ife but Benin soon developed its own matchless beauty and technique. The use of bronze was reserved for the King and

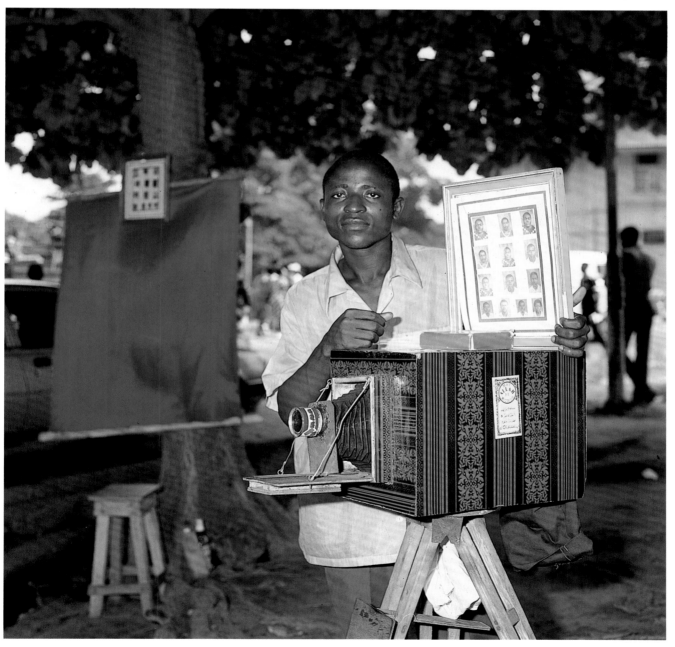

Street photographer in Lagos

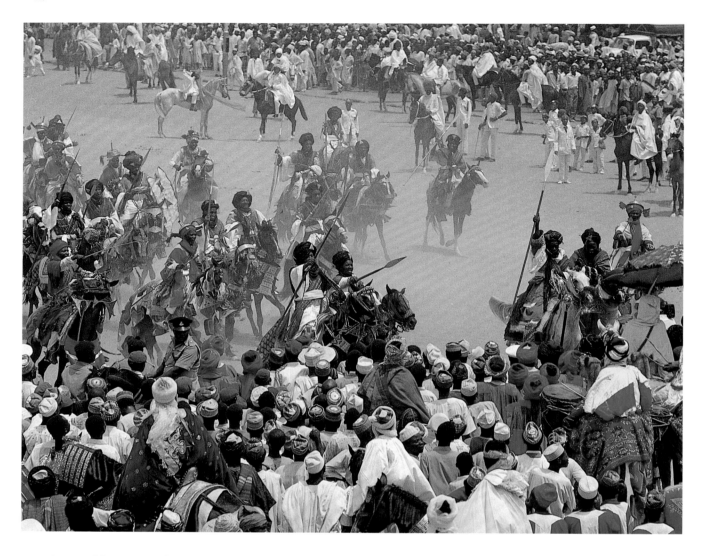

precious gifts were also commissioned for favoured visitors and subjects. The beauty and elegance of the bronzework is breathtaking, with many figures bearing the decoration of their office; elaborate plaques and superb animals were also produced at this period. The art of Benin attracted the early wonder and attention of European visitors to the area. After the sack of the city by the British punitive expedition in 1897 the finest examples of Benin art were scattered throughout the world to become cherished exhibits in the great collections of the West. The fame of Benin throughout the world has been aided by the amount of knowledge and first-hand reports available. Portuguese traders first reached the area in 1485, to trade firearms and guns for ivory, textiles and spices. The prestige and power of the kings of Benin impressed foreign visitors and the accompanying wealth in turn attracted the

trading interests of Europeans. Internal disputes and the decline of many traditional trading structures finally weakened the integrity of the Benin Empire.

Whilst much of the art of Nigeria has come from cultures and civilisations centred on the forest areas of the south, the north of the country has for more than a thousand years been influenced by its neighbours across the great desert in North Africa. This influence has seen most noticeably the steady and progressive influence of Islam to become the dominant religion of the area. The process of supplanting traditional religions was a slow one, and is matched by the progress of Christianity (although at a much later date) in this respect in the south.

The remarkable Saifawa dynasty ruled in an area centred on northeast Nigeria based on Kanem-Borno for almost a thousand years, from 1085 to 1846. At its peak the area controlled extended to beyond Lake Chad. The two main phases which lasted until the 16th century are usually known as the Kanuri empires. These ancient kingdoms had the advantage of contact through trans-Saharan trade as well as from the institutions of Islam, of which the Hajj was most important. The links with Kanem-Borno and North Africa, as well as Egypt, were of particular value. These ancient kingdoms tended to develop vigorous and effective political administrations based on Islamic precepts, with complementary military and juridical organisations. They were invigorated by the constant movement of travellers, merchants and scholars, and by the movement of people through emigration, war and marriage. There was a constant procession of caravans and embassies across the vast region of the empire. The growth of the religious classes, as the *ulema*, saw the development of a scholastic tradition, an appreciation of the power of literacy and the growth of patronage.

opposite: **Durbar, Katsina Sallah**

below: **Part of the parade at the Katsina Sallah, the yearly festival to celebrate 'Id**

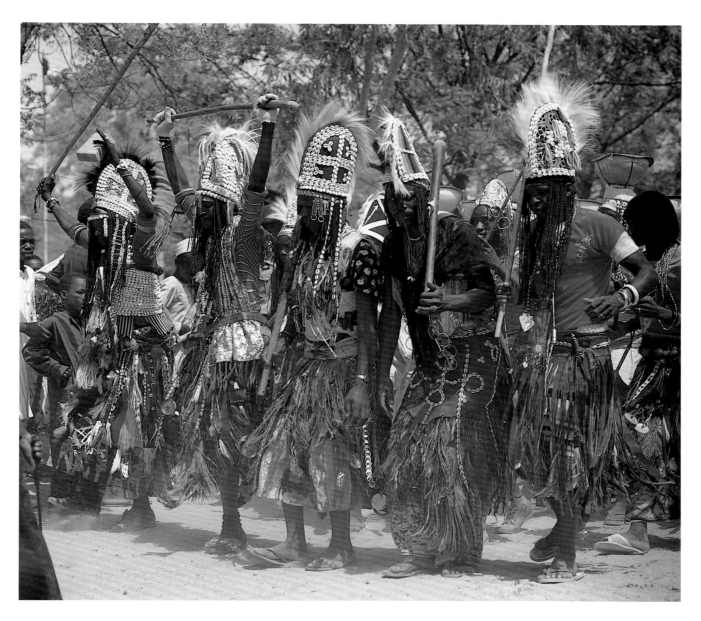

-44-

During the 19th century the ancient empire faced attacks by the Fulani who were fired by the reforming religious zeal of Usuman dan Fodio and his followers. It buckled under such attacks, and the inherent weaknesses led to many internal revolts and the emergence of new leaders. In the latter part of the century Mahdist leaders fleeing from the Sudan gained a large measure of control. To combat this situation, the assistance of the British was sought.

To the west of the Kanuri empire were the lands of the various Hausa tribes, which during the 19th century were dominated by the *Jihad* of Usuman dan Fodio. This religious reformer of great piety and energy proclaimed his *Jihad* in 1804 and came to establish the Sokoto Caliphate. His reforms appealed to the majority of the area at the time and his success was aided by the instability of his adversaries. The Hausa tribes formed various states among

below: Traditional masquerade by the Igbila Moni of Abonnema at Abonnema village in River State

opposite: A musician on horseback at the Katsina Sallah

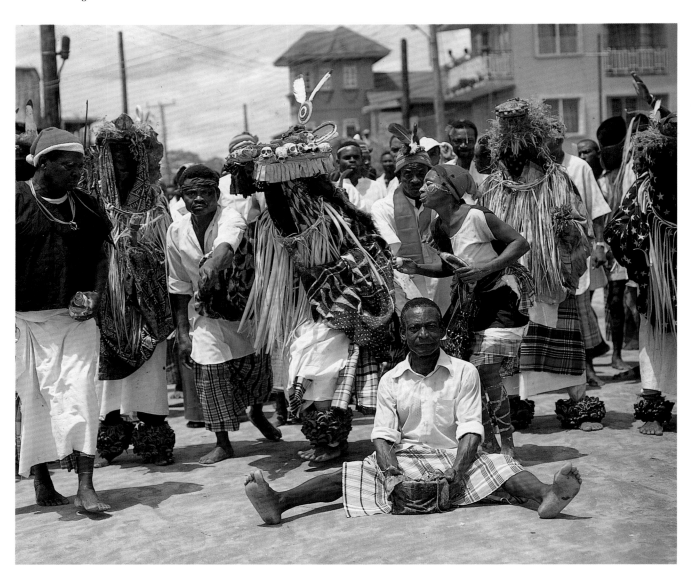

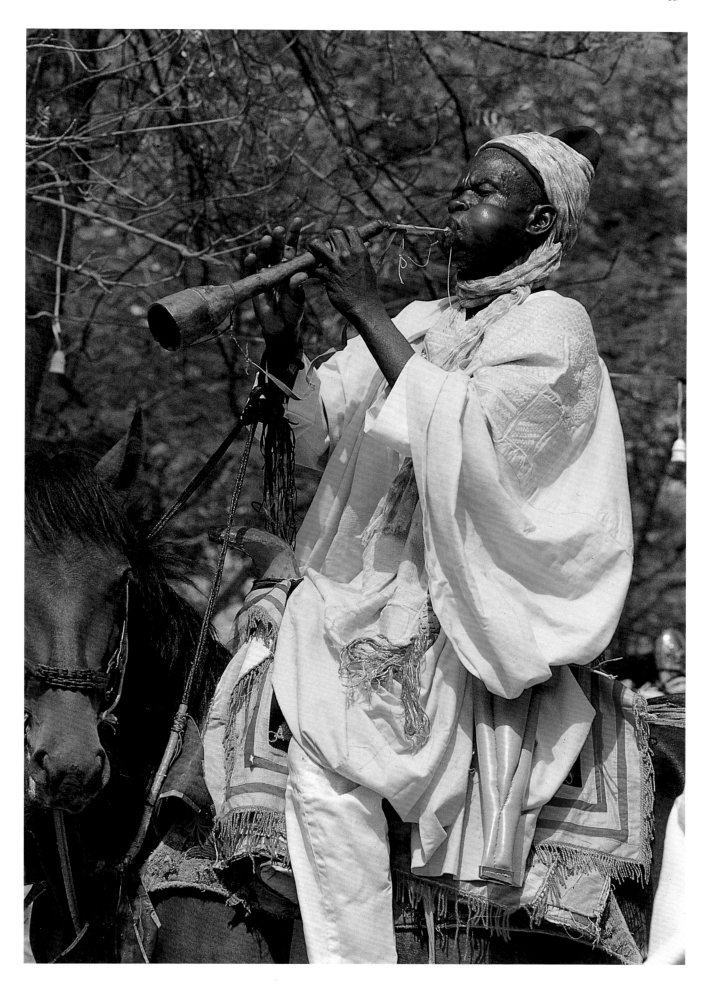

themselves and were held together by a common culture and sense of identity deriving from a common heritage. The Hausa were also responsible for producing their own indigenous artistic traditions. Amongst the most important were the kingdoms based on Zaria, Kano and Katsina. Islam spread among these peoples from the 14th century onwards, mainly as a result of the contacts with their neighbours in the east. Islam and its unifying social and religious structure gave strength to the society, although traditional beliefs were still widely practised.

Usuman dan Fodio derived considerable support from the Fulani, who were skilled, shrewd and reliable, and he initiated political and religious reforms. The Caliphate initially

Chiefs preparing for a chieftancy ceremony at the Oba's palace at Ile-Ife, Oyo State

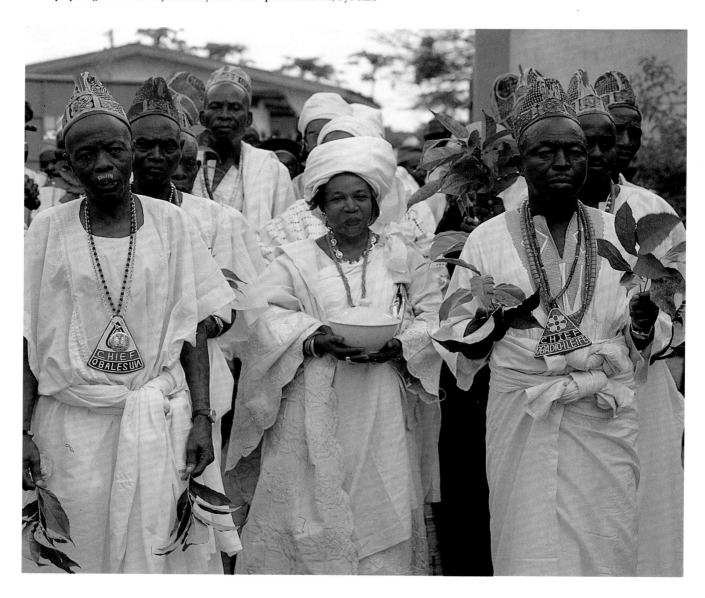

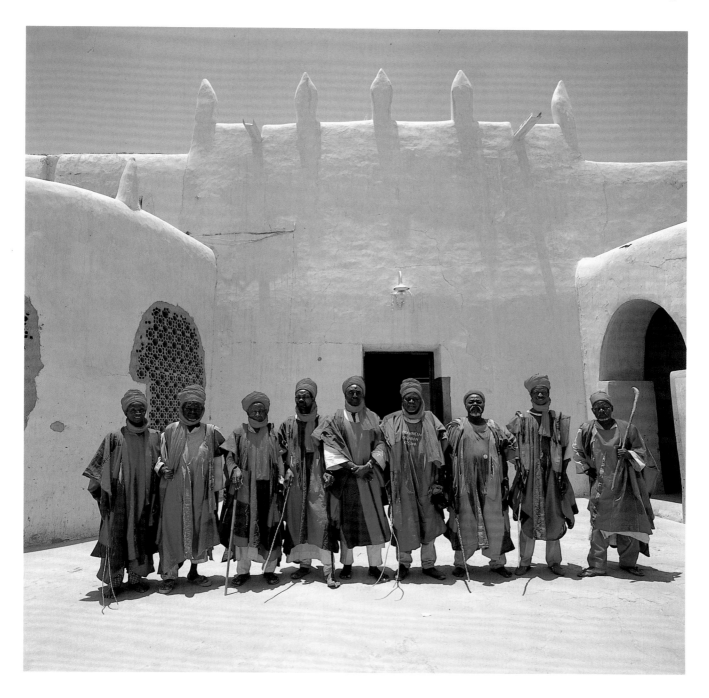

Dongari (Emir's bodyguards) at the Emir's palace in Katsina

offered in a troubled region a stability from which the economy began to thrive. The law and the structure of society were reformed to reflect Islamic precepts. The power of the Caliphate extended far and wide to disrupt adjacent areas, and, for example, put pressure on the Yoruba to the south. In due course the very size of the Caliphate caused problems of control for the central authority, as did the rivalry of Borno and the rapacity of internal opportunists. European interest and influence in the region was also increasing during the 19th century. Eventually it fell to the control of the British, who, under Lugard's administration, created the Northern Protectorate around Kano and Sokoto in 1903.

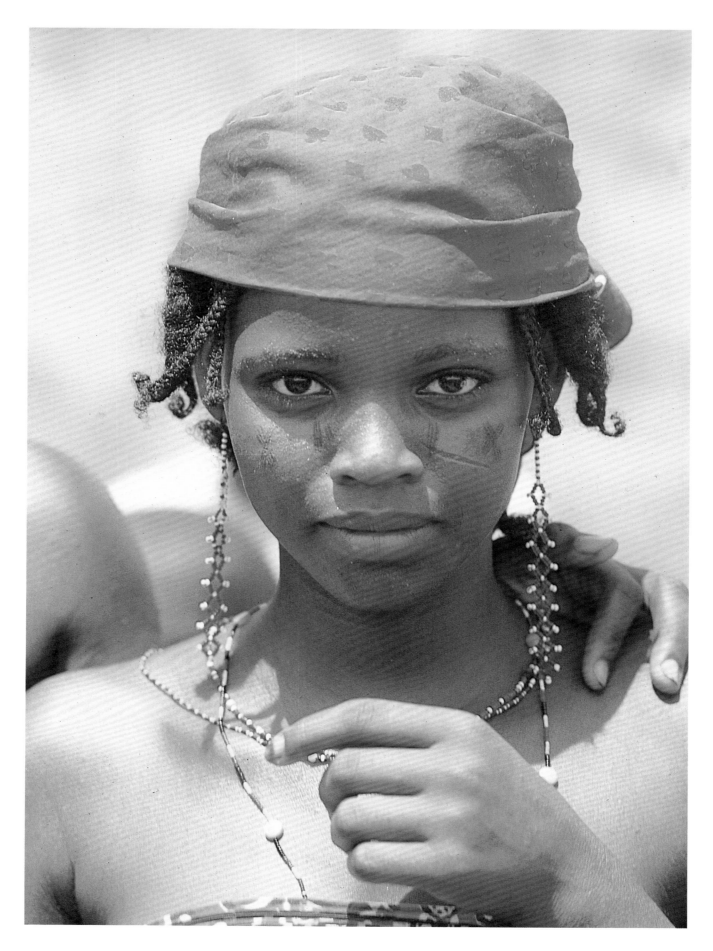

Young Fulani woman, Obudu in Cross River State

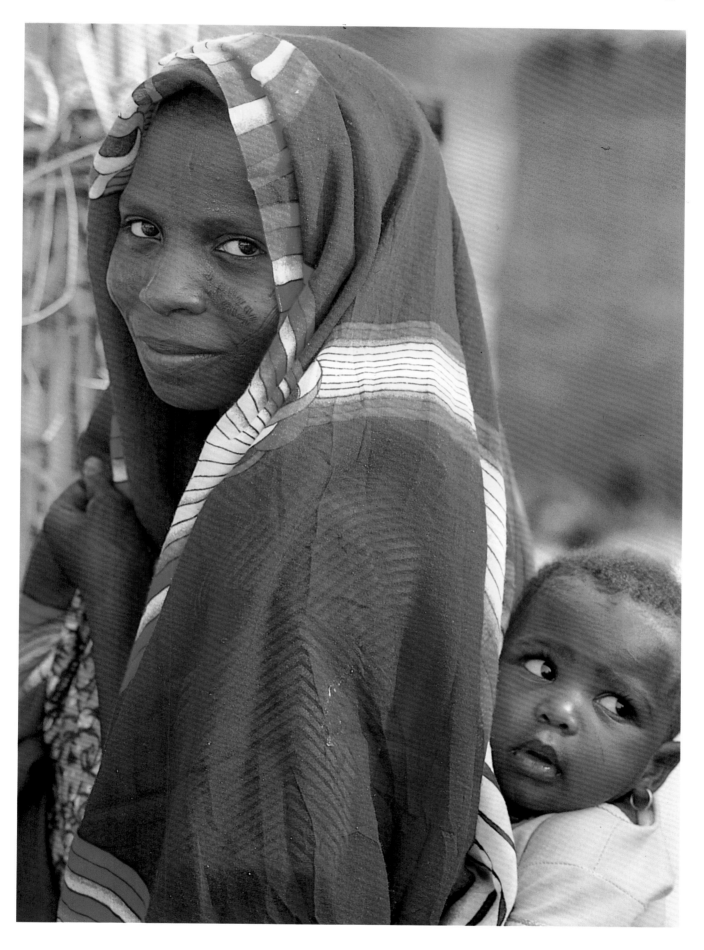

Hausa mother and child, Gobirawa village, Kaduna State

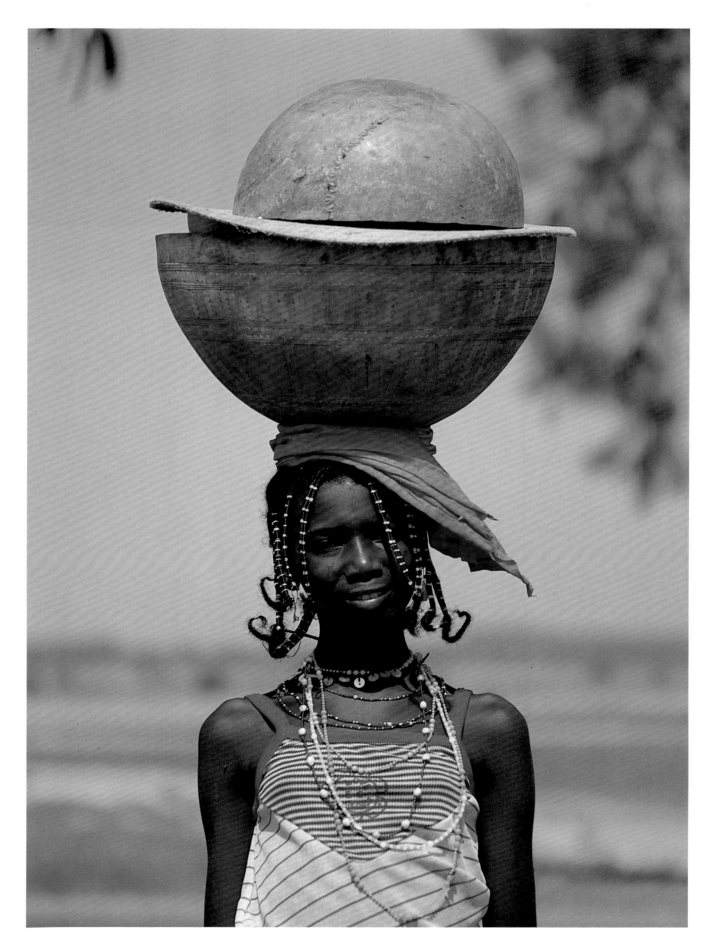

Fulani girl with calabash, Plateau State

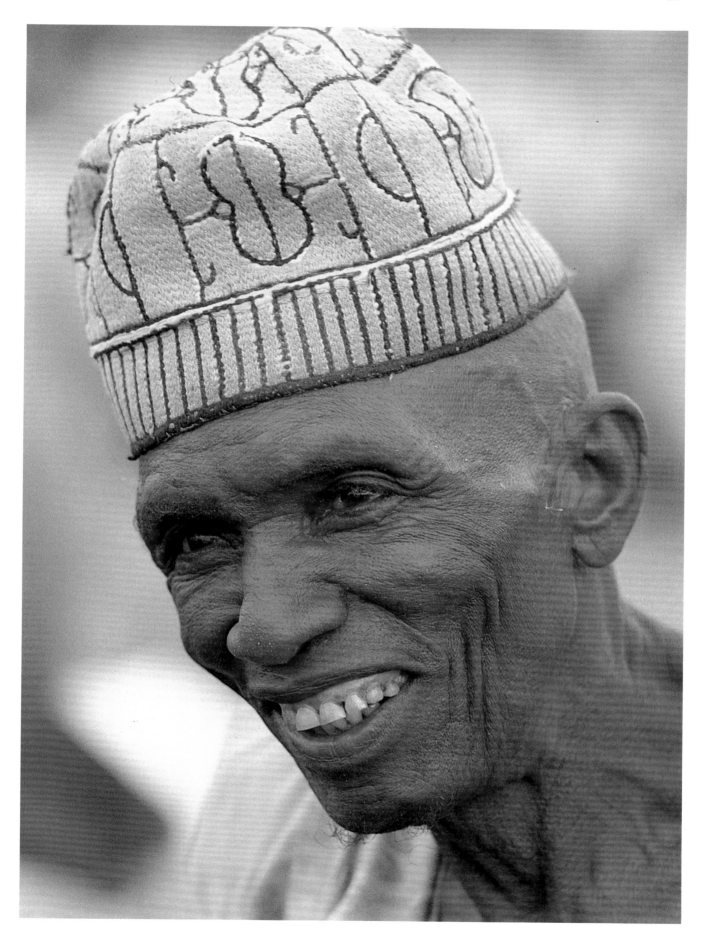

Hausa man, Kano

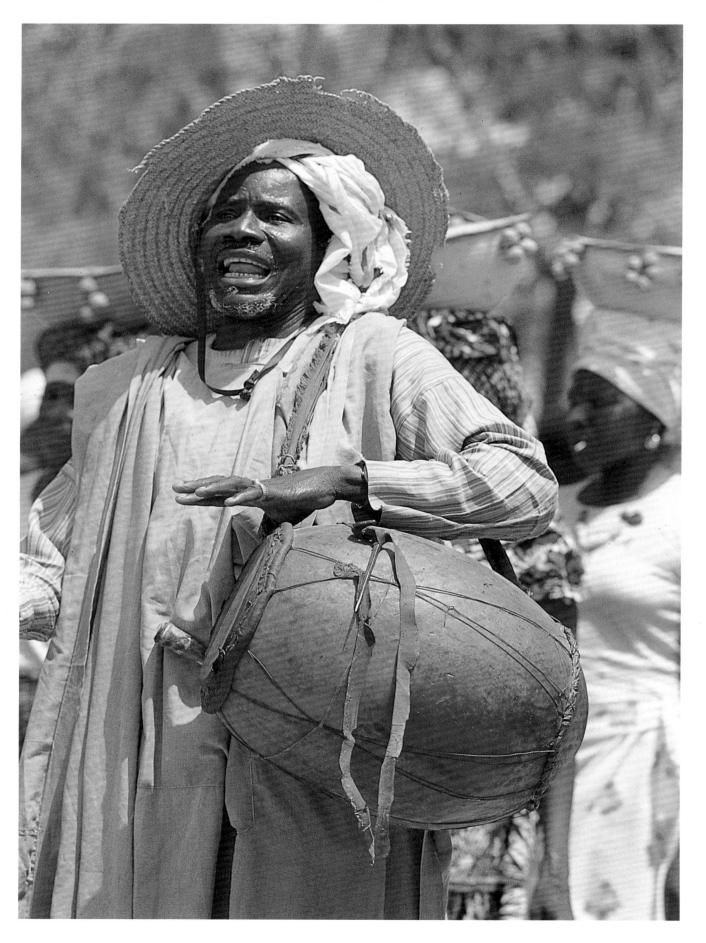

A drummer at the Katsina Sallah

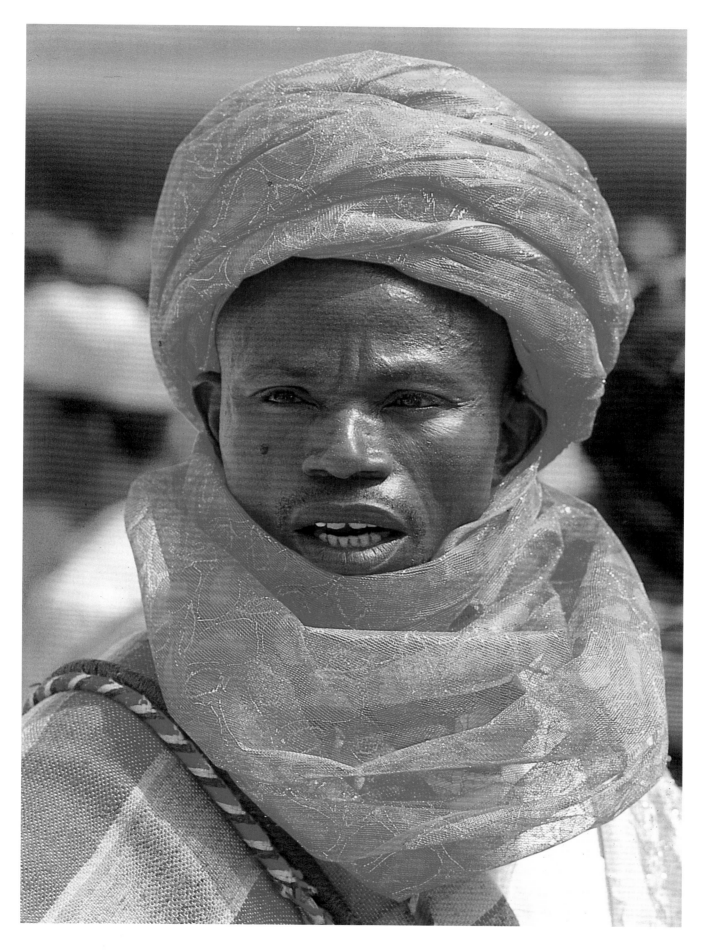

A young man taking part in the Katsina Sallah

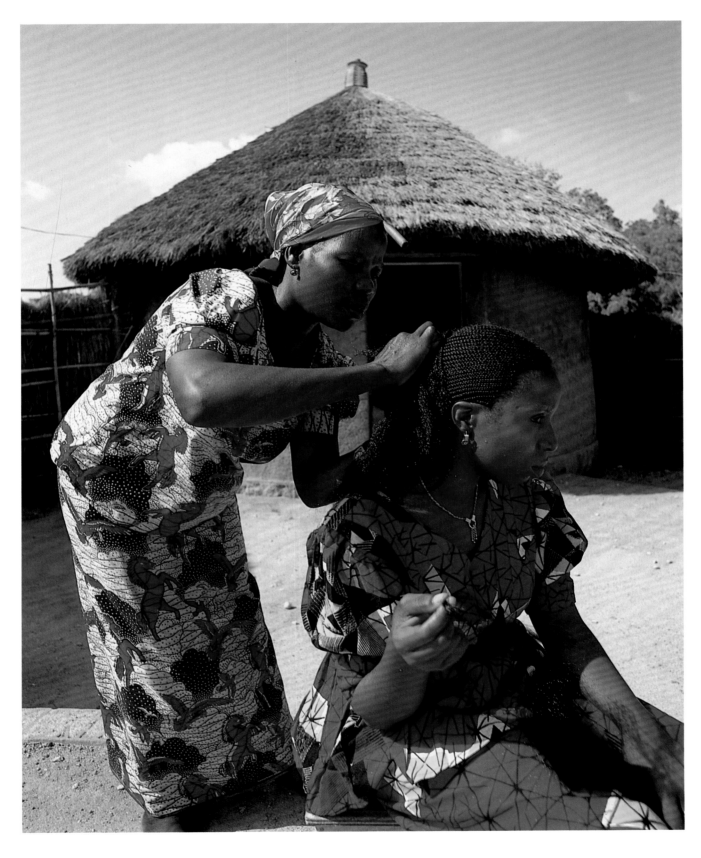

The art of hair plaiting in Jos, Plateau State

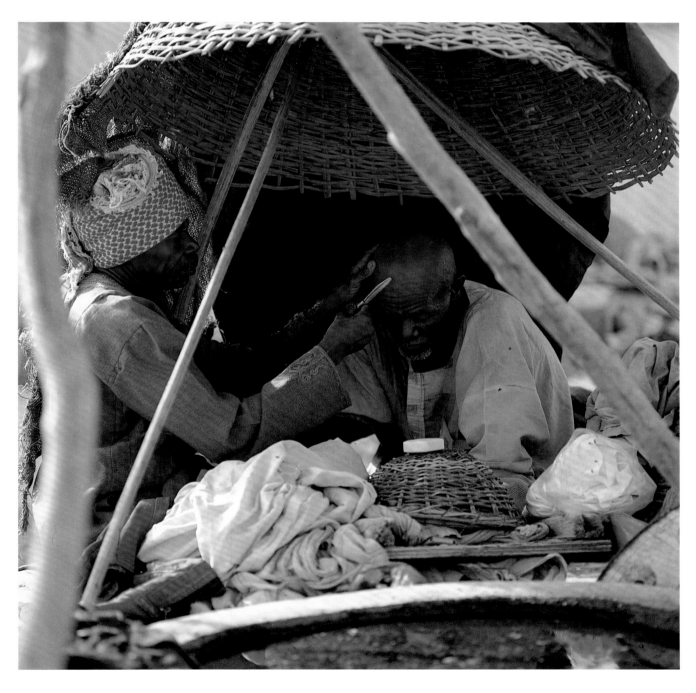

Barber in Kano

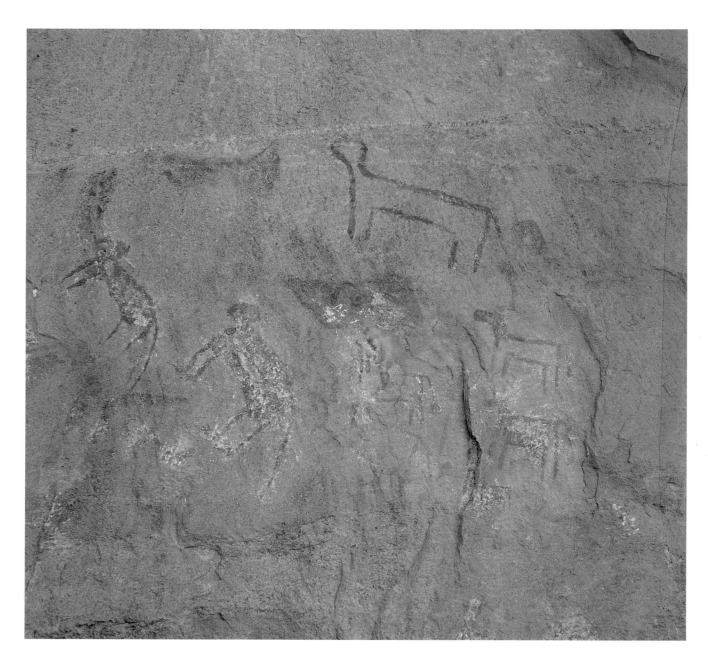

Geji rock paintings, Bauchi State

ART AND CULTURE

THE great variety of Nigerian artistic achievements is apparent not only in artefacts from the past but also in the multiplicity of high quality works being produced today. There are names famous worldwide in the disciplines of literature and music: names such as Wole Soyinka, the 1986 winner of the Nobel Prize for Literature, and others like Chinua Achebe, Cyprien Ekwensi, Amos Tutuola and the renowned musicians Fela Anikulapo-Kuti and King Sunny Ade. Achievements in other areas, both those with renowned exponents and those stemming from a more anonymous communal background as befits African tradition, deserve mention.

Musa Yola, for instance, has excelled in the art of painting, applying most of his work to the decoration of buildings and houses, a technique which saw a veritable explosion of artists between the 1940s and 1970s. Chequerboard patterns and flower motifs are popular decorations in this kind of art, although Musa Yola specialises as much in human figures, the representation of buildings and objects of modern industrial life. Another painter to gain wide recognition for his work on board and paper is Mike Irrifere, a member of the important Uli school of painters, whose work deals with the human figure within its social context. Other prominent Nigerian artists are Jimoh Buraimoh, renowned for his bead paintings, Bruce Onobrakpeya for his monographs of prints and painting, and Ben Enwonwu for his excellent sculptures, have all attained international recognition for their works. More communal arts encompass disciplines like woodcarving, much of which is accomplished on household articles such as stools and food bowls, pottery both for decorative and practical use, and metalwork, which for a long time has been an art of great importance in many areas of Nigeria. Leatherwork is particularly important in the Northern part of Nigeria. Dyeing, raffia work, weaving, ceramics, glass beads and basketry are also worthy of mention, and not least the art of building as expressed by indigenous architecture.

Calabash decoration is one of the distinctive Nigerian arts: calabashes, or gourds, ranging from those large enough to be used as rafts by fishermen to those small enough to be used as delicate salt shakers, are prepared first by cleaning out the ripe fruit and then worked on with a variety of tools, from saws to knives and scrapers. In the North, calabashes are still commonly used as milk containers and in other areas as grain storage utensils.

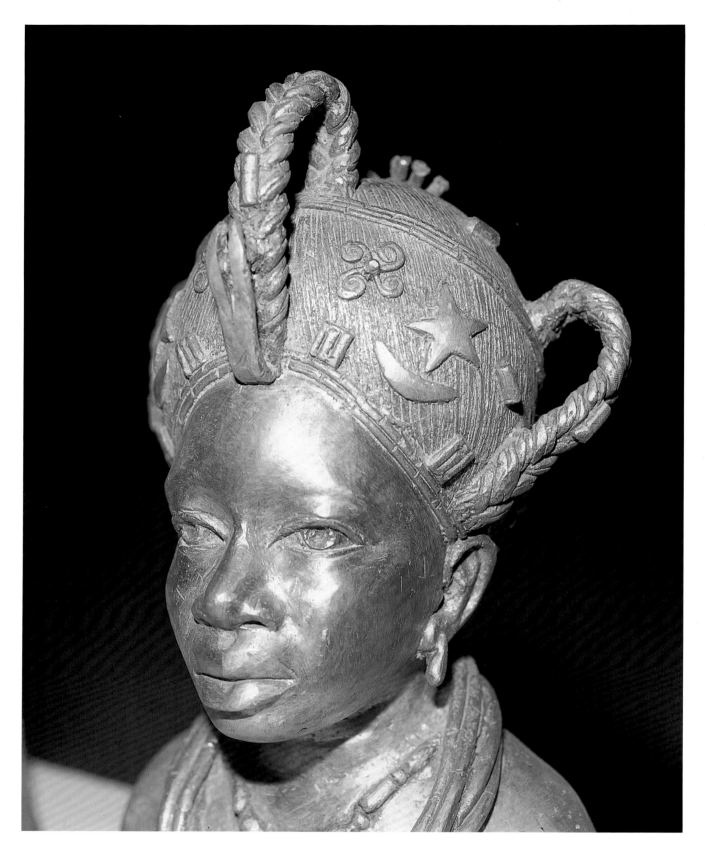

Bronze head figurine, Minna Museum

A 16th century bronze plaque depicting an oba and attendants
celebrating a war victory in ceremonial garb, Benin Museum

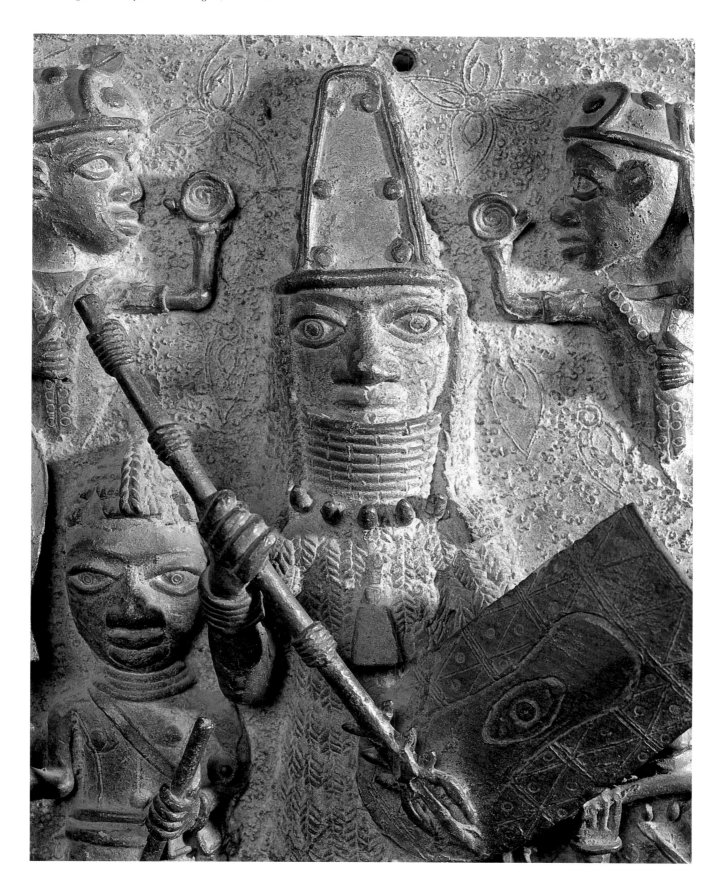

Detail of a Nupe pot with lizard motif

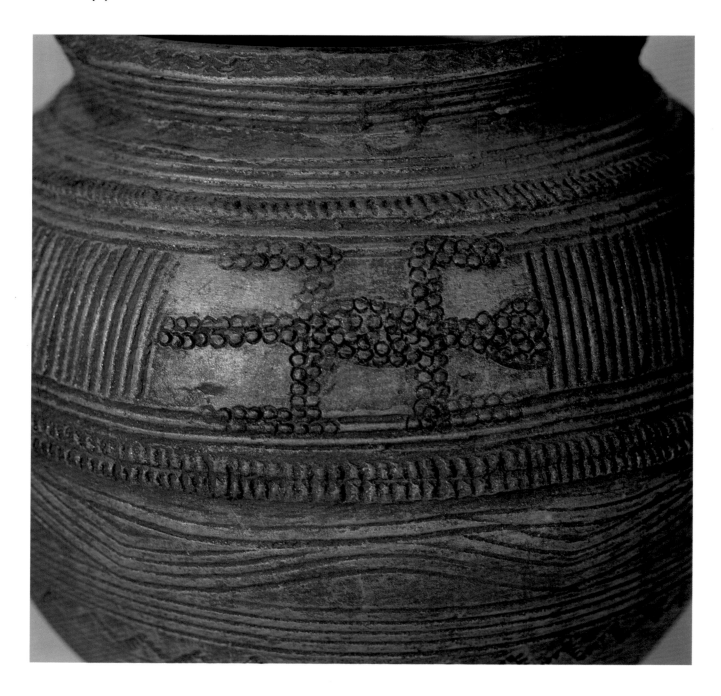

Nupe wedding pot

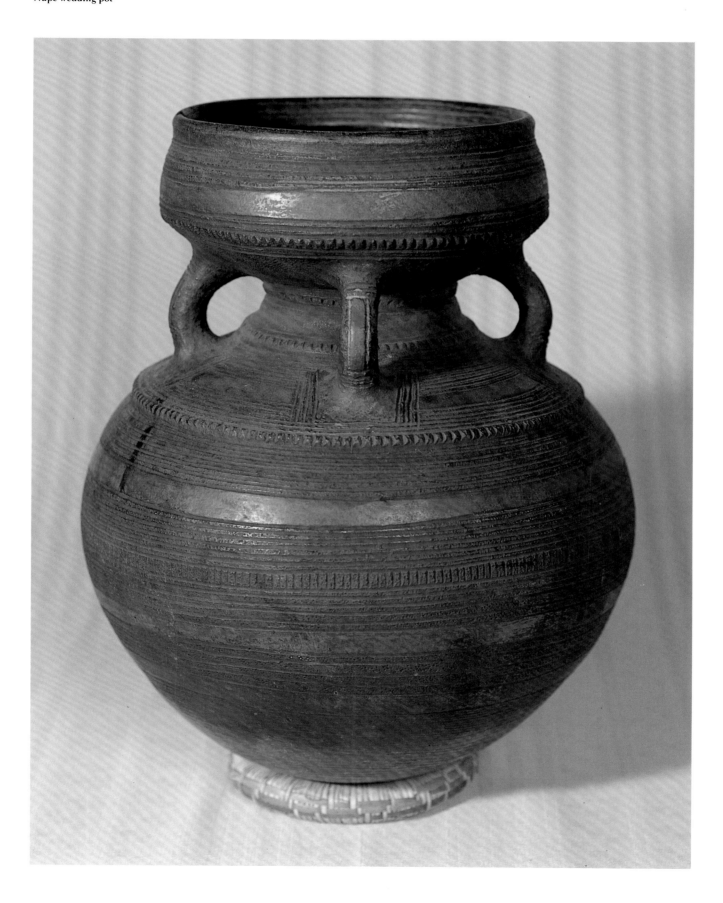

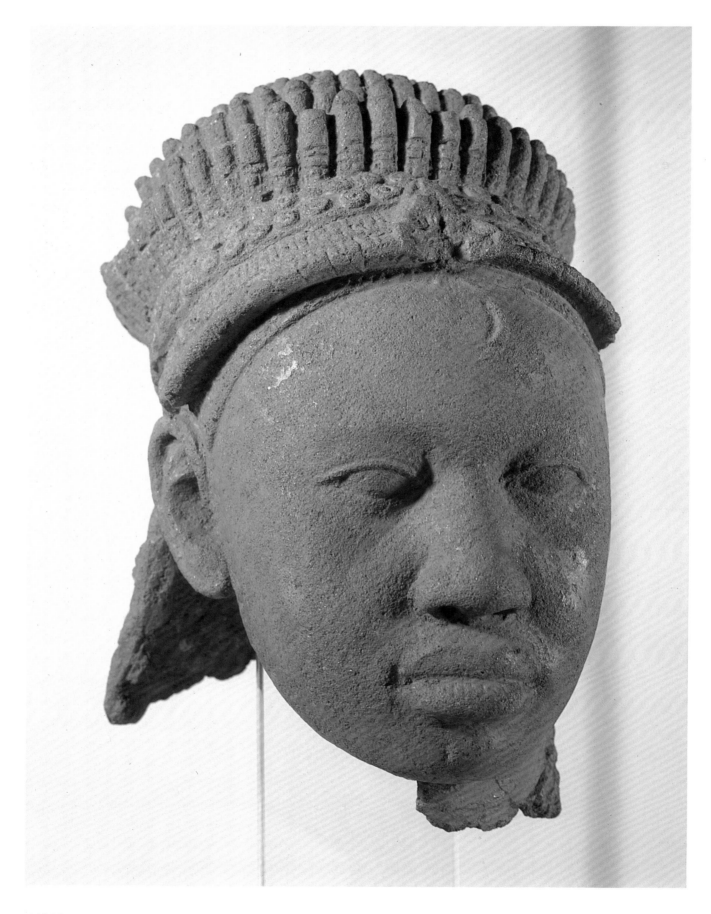

12th/13th century terracotta, Ife. The five-tiered beaded crown indicates
that this head, originally part of a full-length figure, represents a queen. It
is the most elaborate terracotta yet found in Ife. National Museum, Lagos.

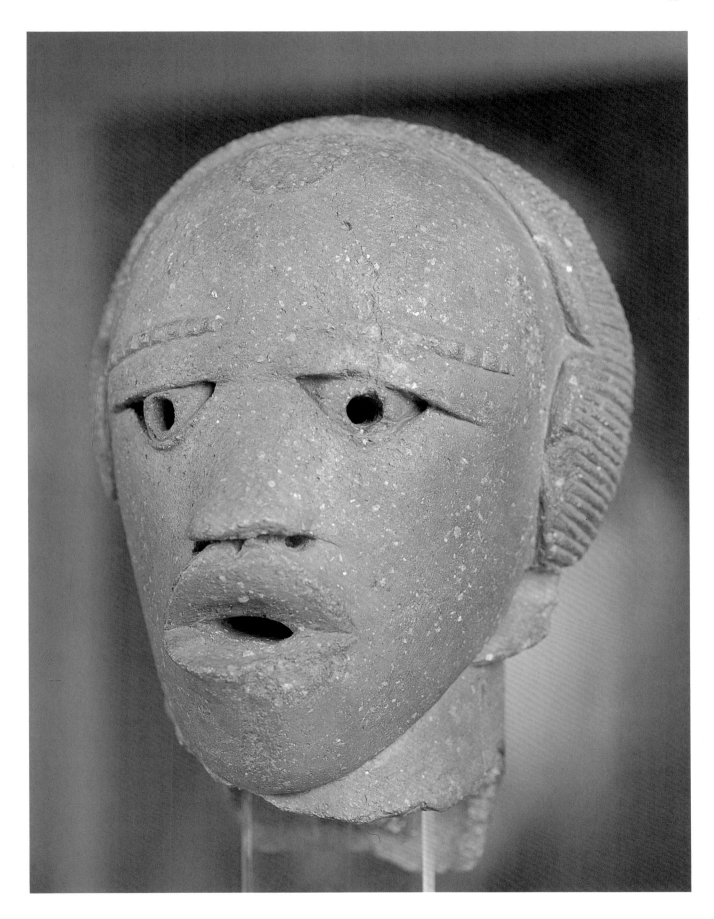

The Jemaa Head, 5th century BC Nok terracotta. One of the two heads found at Tsauni Camp, Jemaa, in 1943 which convinced Bernard Fagg that there was an unknown culture of considerable antiquity in the area around Nok. National Museum, Lagos.

Food Bowl made from carved wood, Kano Museum

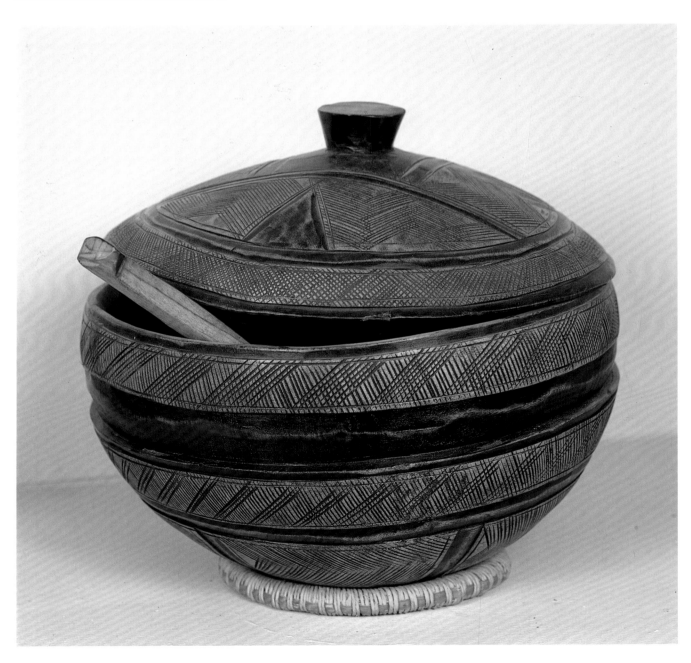

Wood mask of the Ekpo cult, Benin Museum

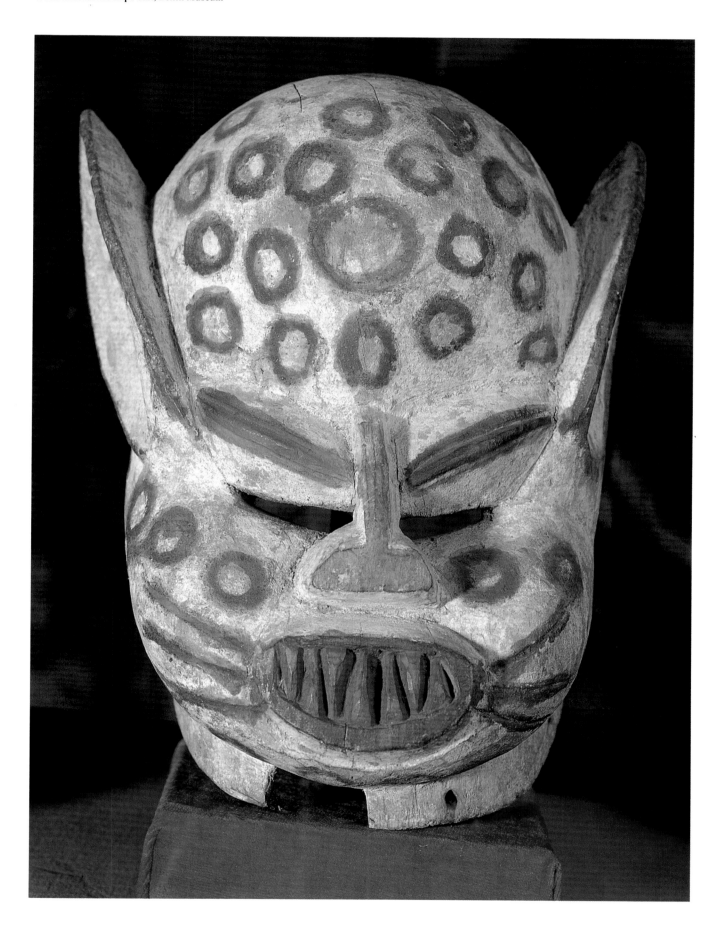

Gelede mask from Meko, Jos Museum

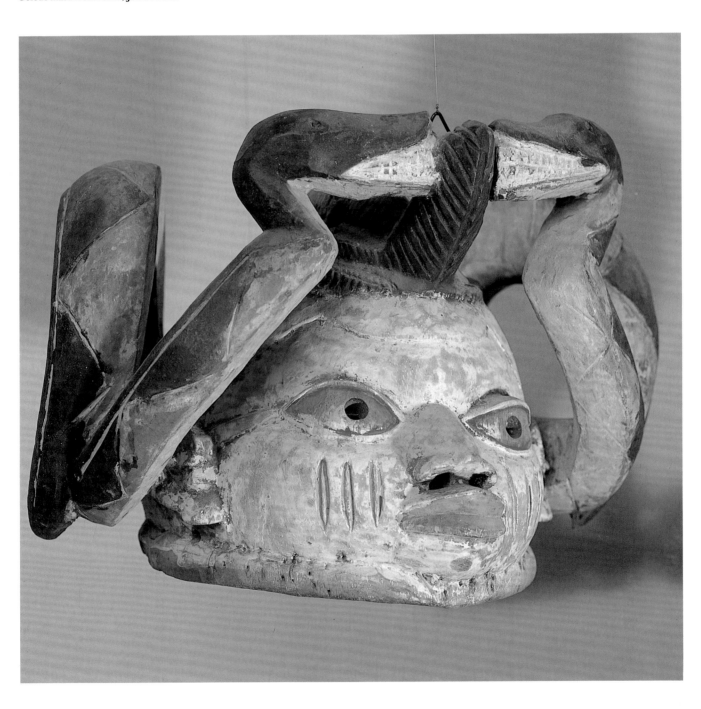

Jarawa pottery in the Jos Museum

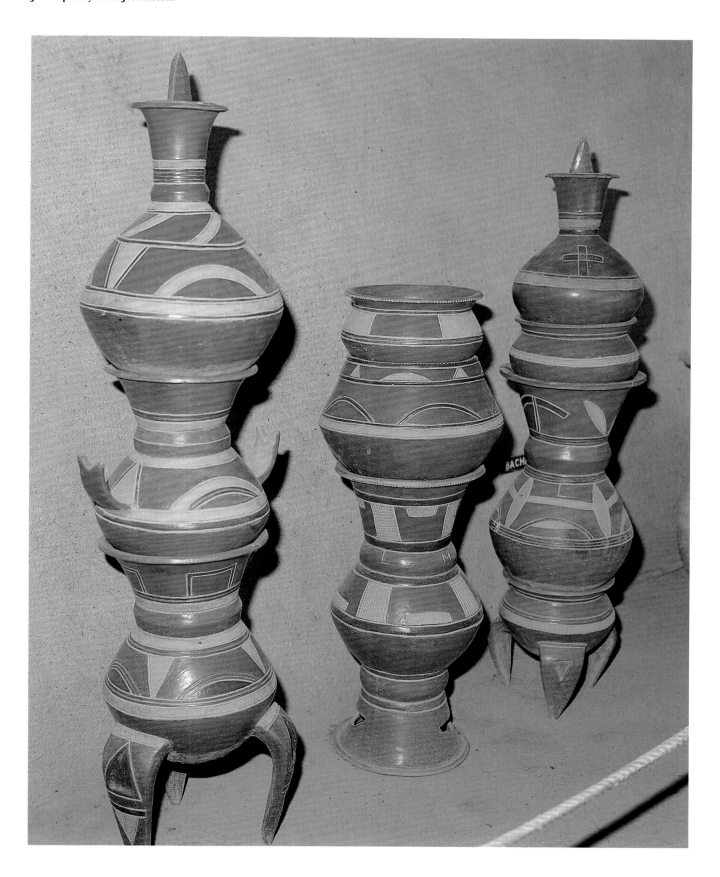

Roped Pot on a stand. 9th/10th century leaded bronze, from Igbo-Isaiah,
Igbo-Ukwu. The stand on this elaborate casting, excavated in the remains of
a storehouse, perhaps reflects the still prevalent tradition that sacred water
should not touch the earth before it is used in ritual ceremonies.
National Museum, Lagos.

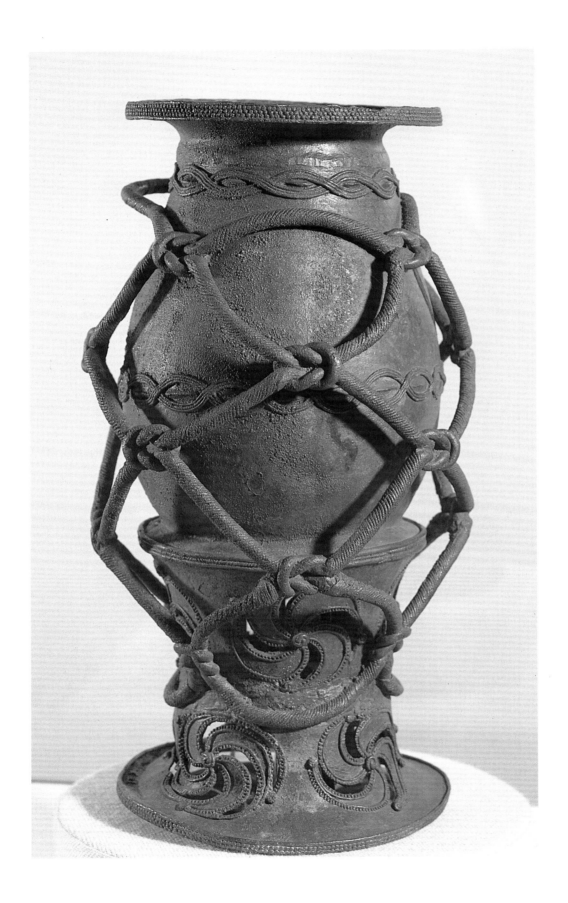

Traditional weaving in Paiko village, Niger State

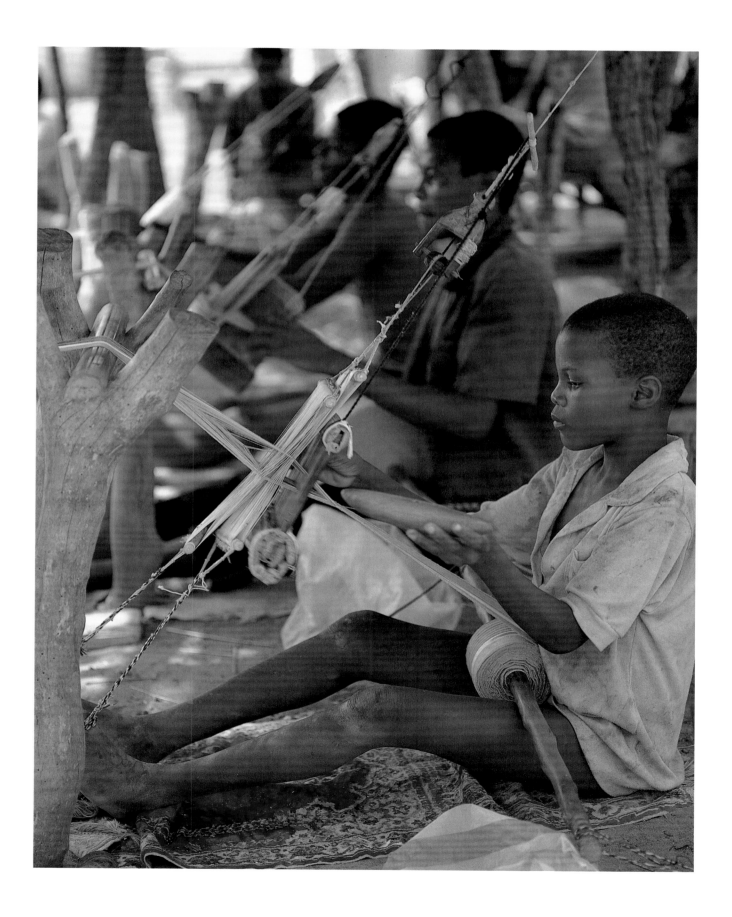

below: **The Naruguta Pottery in Plateau State**

opposite: **Display of pottery skills in Paiko village, Niger State**

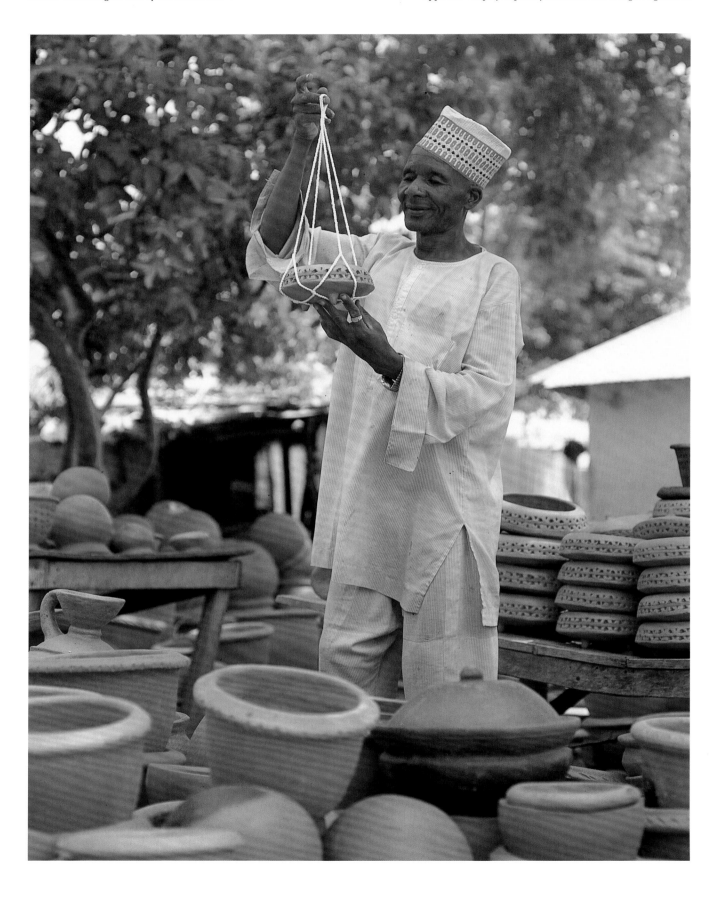

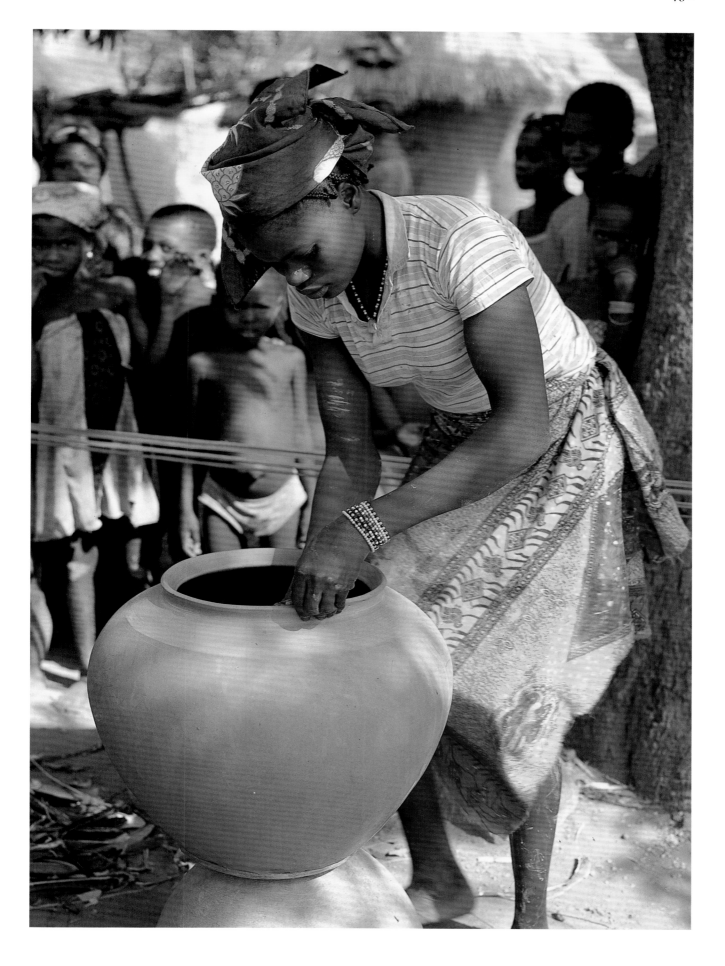

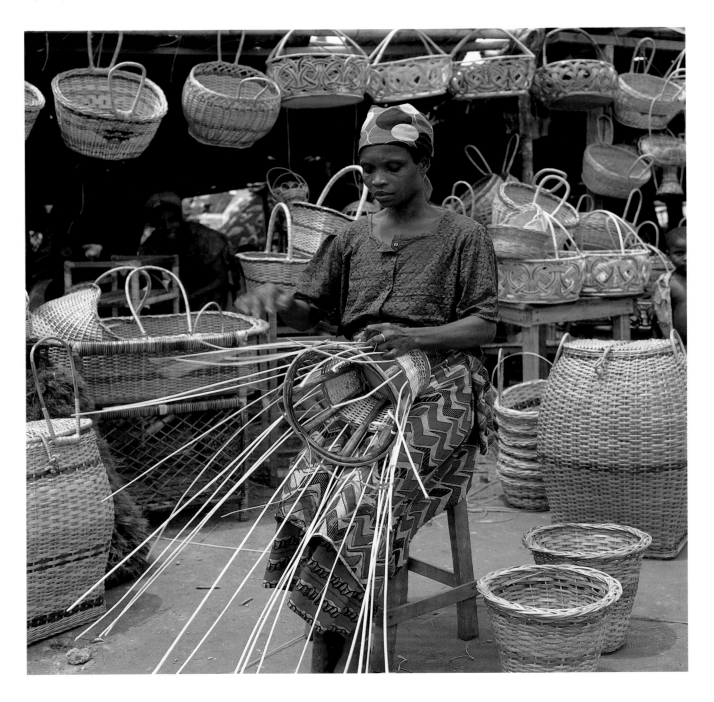

A basketworker in Lagos

Adire print cloth from Abeokuta, Ogun State. Based on an original design
for the jubilee of King George V and Queen Mary, 1935

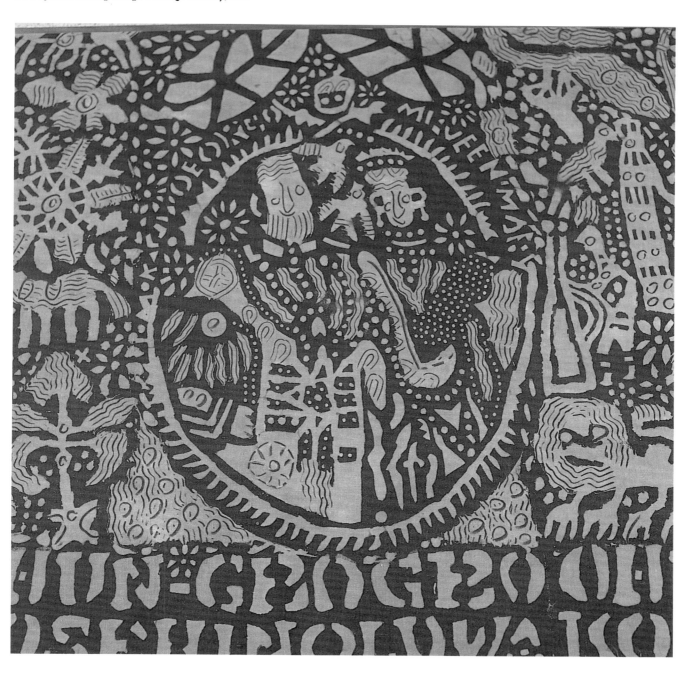

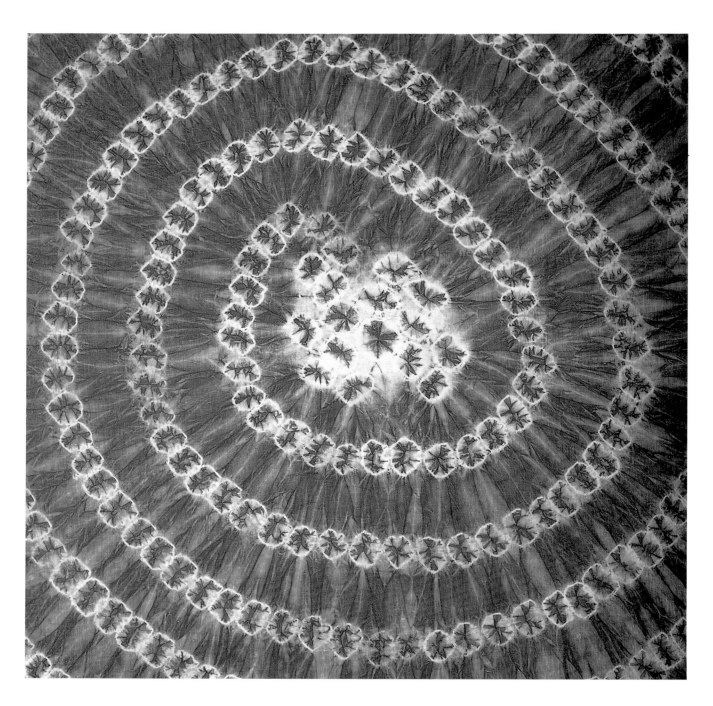

Tie dye, Kano Museum

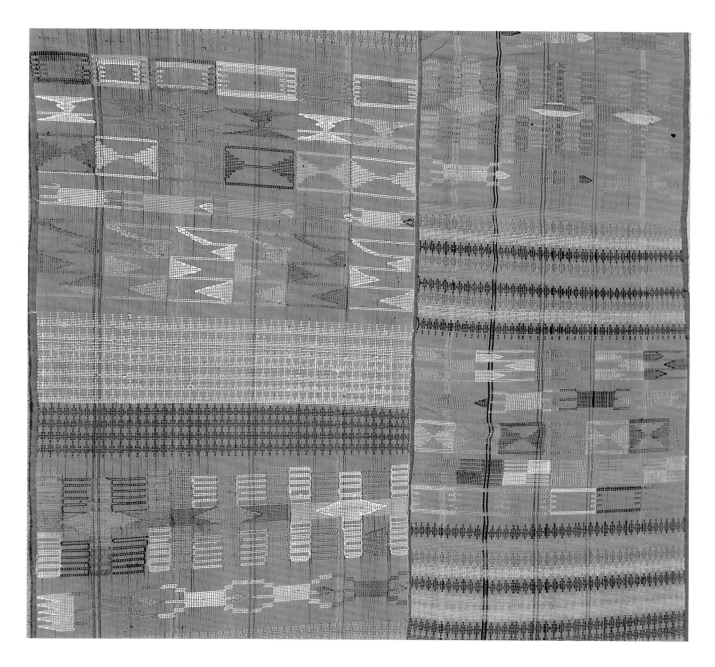

Nupe cloth from Bida, with an Akwete pattern

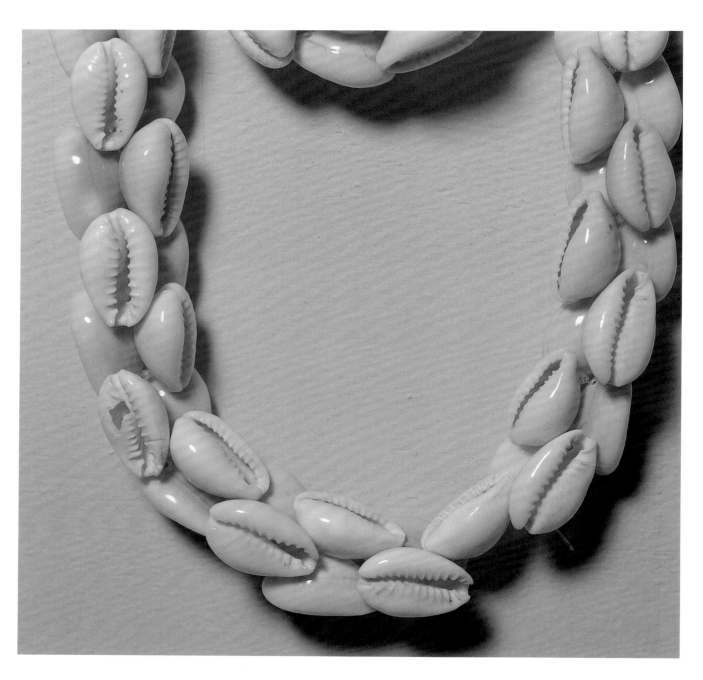

Cowrie necklace, Kano Museum. Cowrie shells were traditionally used as a form of currency.

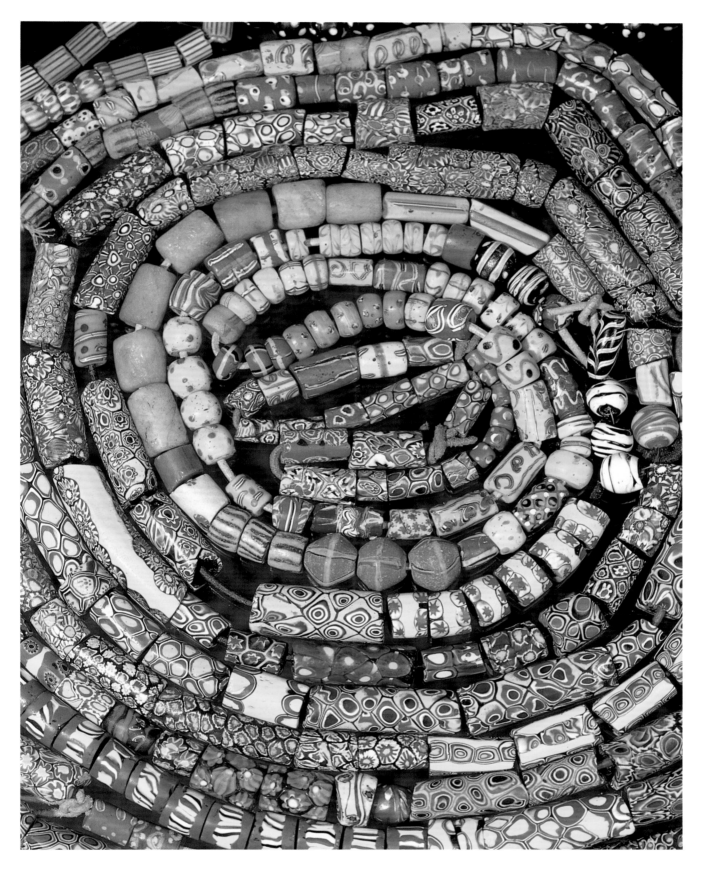

Beads

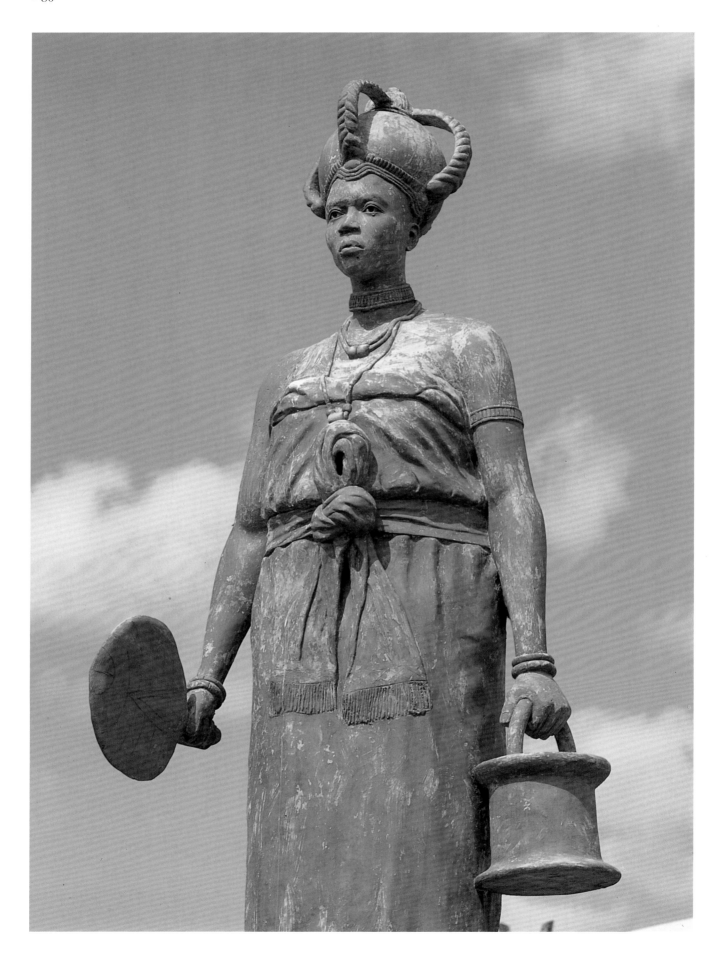

opposite: Statue of Mother Africa, outside the National Museum, Lagos

below: The National Theatre, Lagos

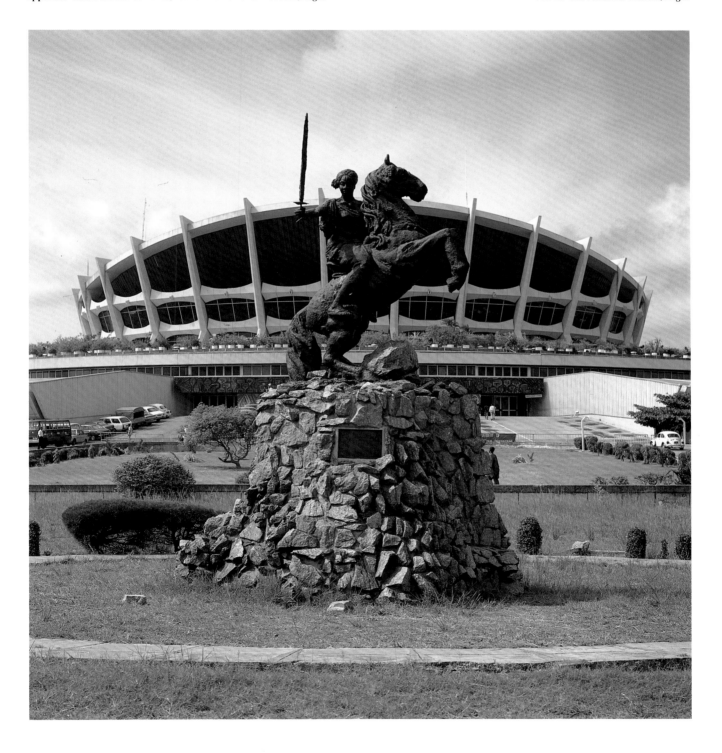

FESTAC AND THE NATIONAL THEATRE

The reputation of Nigeria was enhanced worldwide in the cultural sphere during the 1970s when preparations were set in train for the second African festival of arts and culture (FESTAC). The building of housing estates was begun in Lagos in 1973 which was later to be used for accommodation during the Festival. The National Theatre complex at Iganmu, Lagos, was built in 1976 and served as the venue for the FESTAC activities. FESTAC provided the opportunity to show and promote the enormous variety and achievement of the African and Black peoples within the arts and also confirmed Nigeria's leading place within that cultural spectrum. Its stimulus provided further encouragement for cultural traditions within the country. In 1978 the Centre for Black and African Arts and Civilization (CBAAC) was established as a research centre to continue this advance.

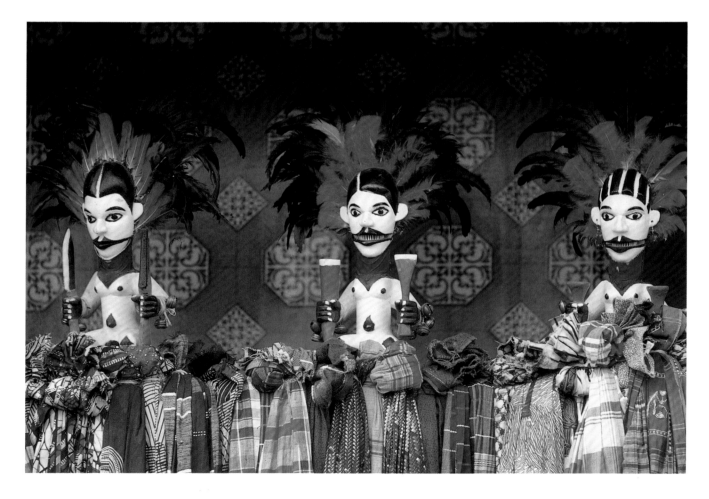

Amanikpo puppet theatre at Gbene-Ue Tai in Rivers State

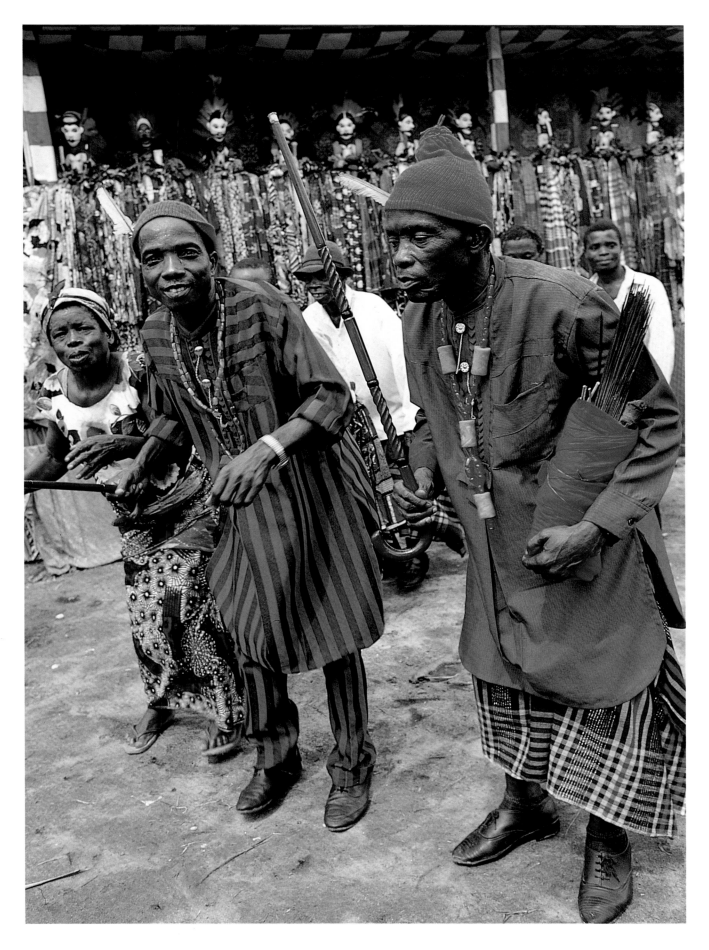

Performers in the Amanikpo puppet theatre, Gbene-Ue Tai, Rivers State

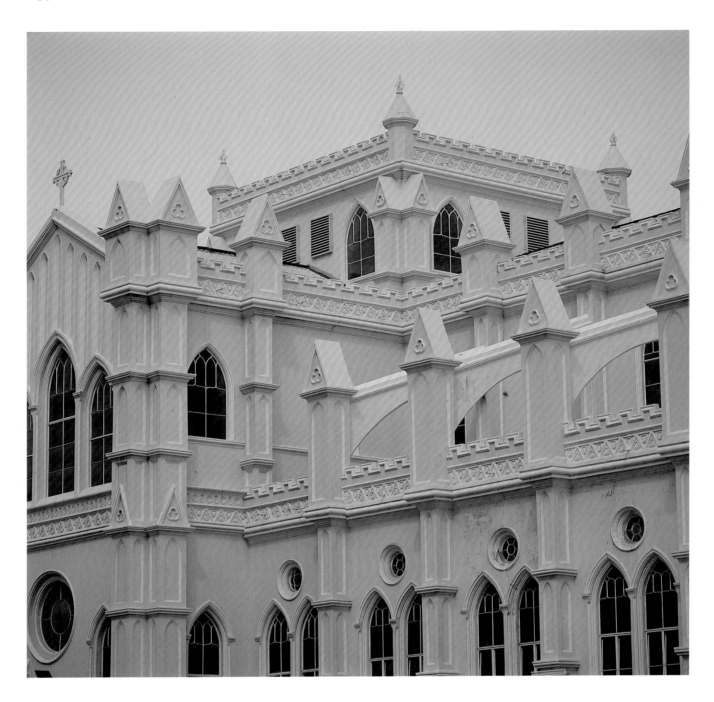

Christ Church Cathedral, Lagos

ARCHITECTURE

NIGERIA'S architecture has developed to suit the prevailing geographical conditions but has often been subject to external influence.

The pre-colonial mud huts with thatched roofs were the earliest form of architecture known in Nigeria. These huts vary in size and shape and exhibit distinctive characteristics according to their geographical location. The dwelling structures of the savannah, for instance, are usually round in shape, low, small and sometimes with conical-shaped thatched roofs. In contrast, larger structures with mud deckings for roofs, instead of the conventional thatched roofings, are found in many towns in the northern states. Some of these structures suggest strong Islamic influence in their designs.

In the rain forest areas of southern Nigeria, houses are also made of mud walls with thatched roofs or corrugated iron sheets, specially designed to resist the heavy rains and also to serve as insulation against the heat of the day. More modern houses built with cement-mixed hollow bricks are generally to be found in larger towns and cities throughout the country. The city walls of Kano and Benin are relics of some of the oldest mud structures in the country.

The colonial administration made extensive use of the rainforest timber (especially in the south) in building construction. The 'raised bungalows' with mud pillar-type foundations and fitted with wooden walls are still to be found in towns like Warri, Ibadan, Jos and Lagos. Closely following these were the British-type colonial town halls with massive pillars. The roofs were high and angular, while the ceilings were made of wood. State House Marina and Mapo Hall, Ibadan, are examples of this architectural type.

Some of the old villa-type structures, usually with small garden forecourts, are still to be found, mostly in the Yaba district of Lagos. They represent another type of architecture previously owned by wealthy Lagosians of the pre-Independence era, as well as Sierra Leonians and Ghanaian settlers in Lagos. Structures built on stilts are commonly found in the riverine areas of Nigeria.

Other foreign influence can be seen in the Brazilian storey-type buildings mostly seen on Lagos Island, some of which have intricate designs and patterns on the walls. Extensive use of iron railings for decoration is also said to have Brazilian origin.

Modern day architecture includes cement-block and concrete structures plus, of course, the high rise office buildings and residential blocks which are found along Broad Street and Marina and the Victoria Island areas of Lagos. Nigeria has been endowed with a great number of modern buildings to meet modern requirements, which buildings stand juxtaposed with earlier styles.

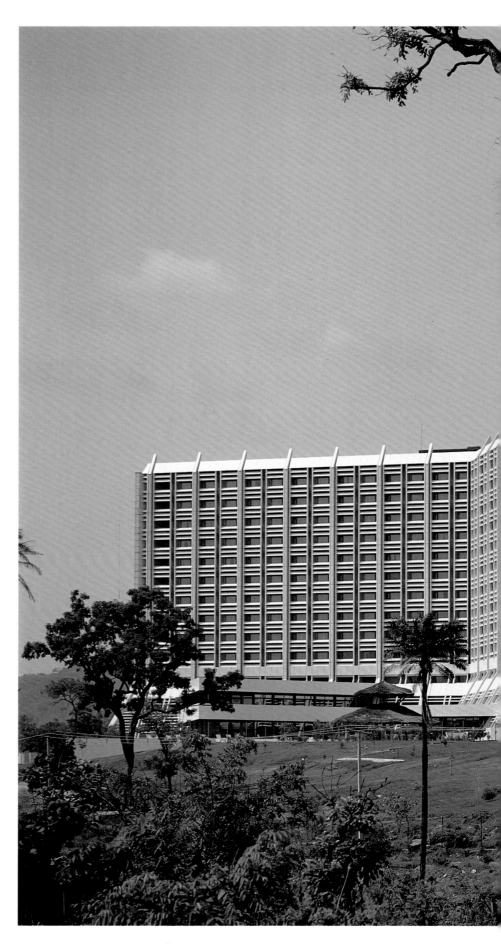

Nicon Noga, the Hilton hotel in Abuja

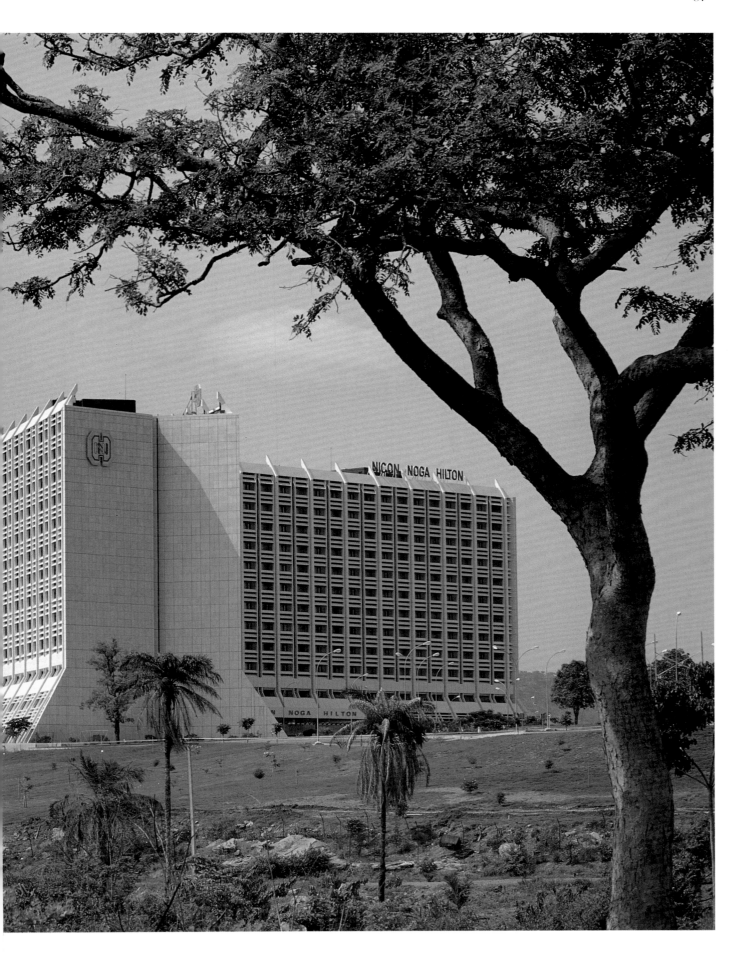

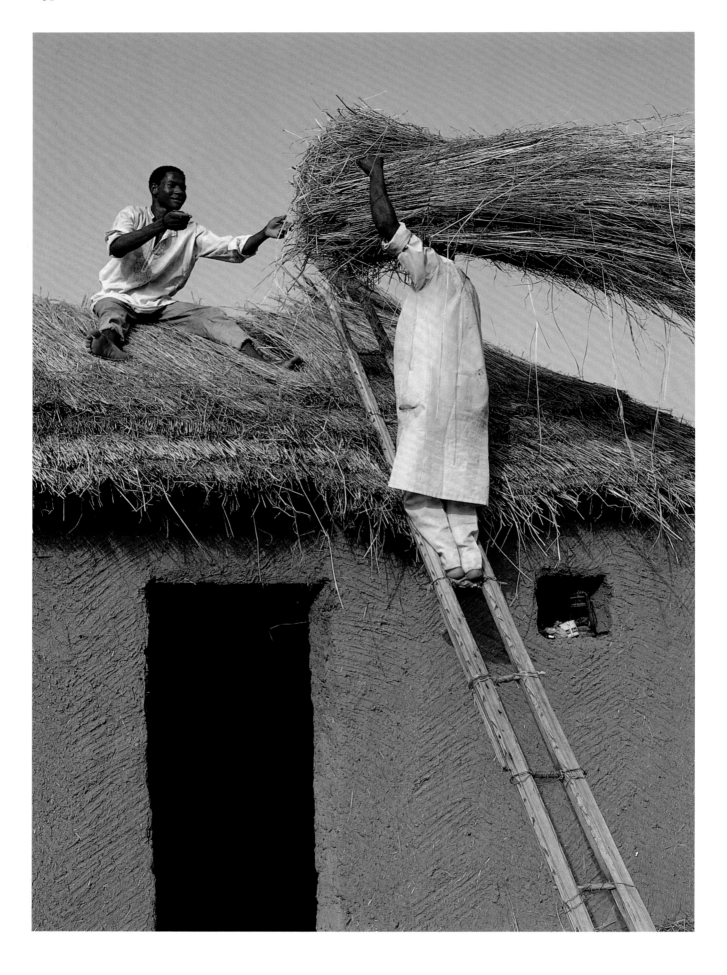

opposite: Roof thatchers at work in Angwuwa Babayi, Kaduna State

below: Old and new architecture – the old Ministry of Communication and the First Bank of Nigeria in Lagos

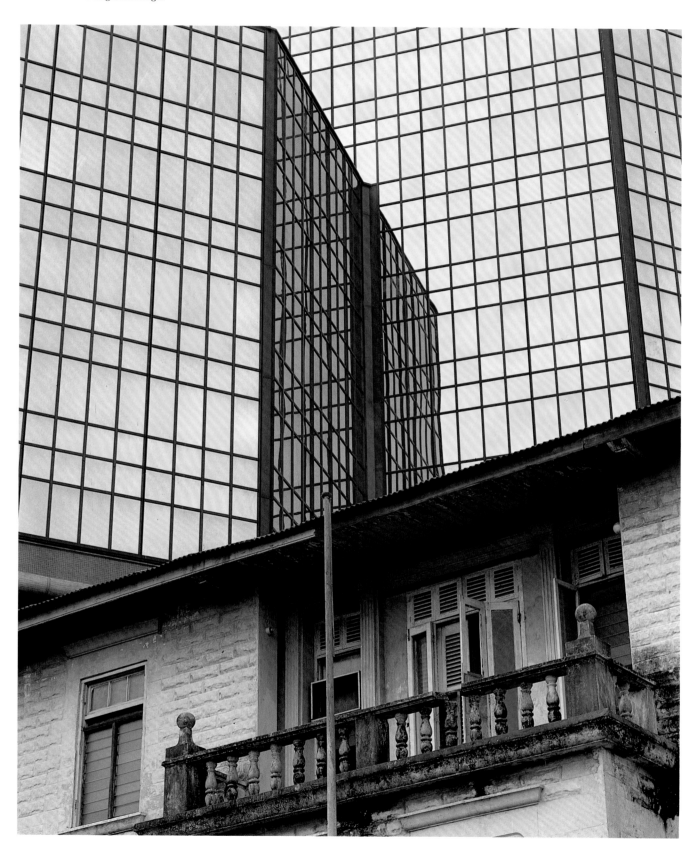

—92—

below: A Nupe women's hut, exhibited in the Jos Museum

opposite: The 300-year-old Gobarau Minaret tower in Katsina, from where according to custom Muslims look towards Mecca

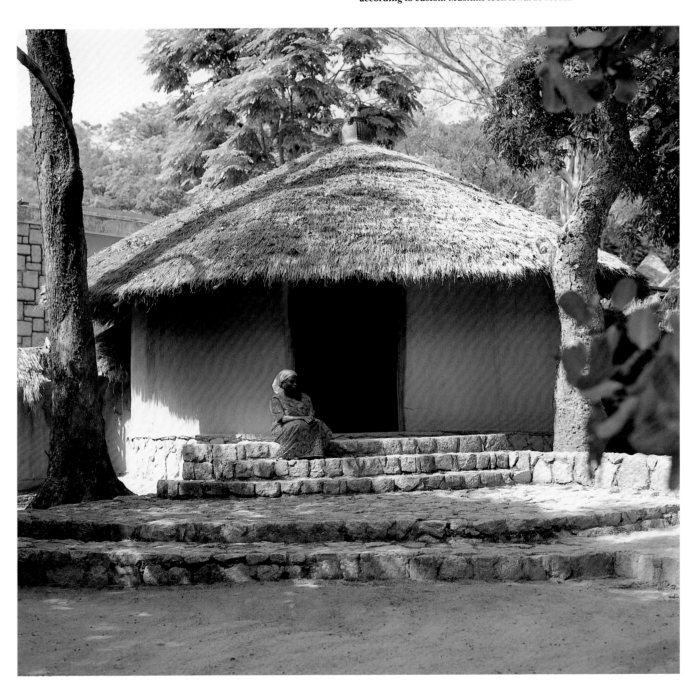

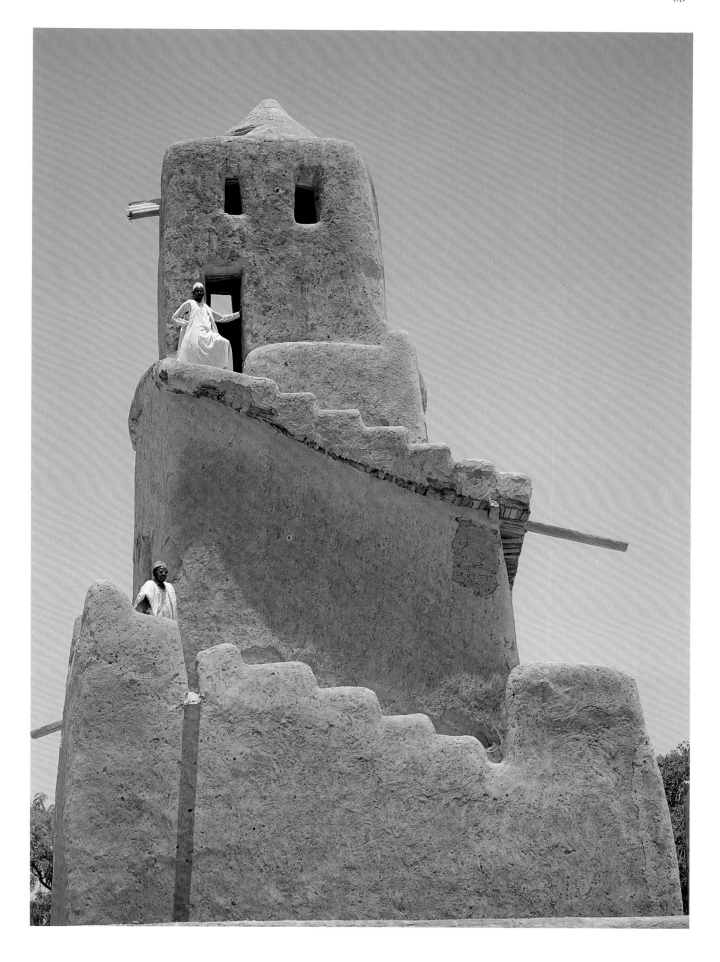

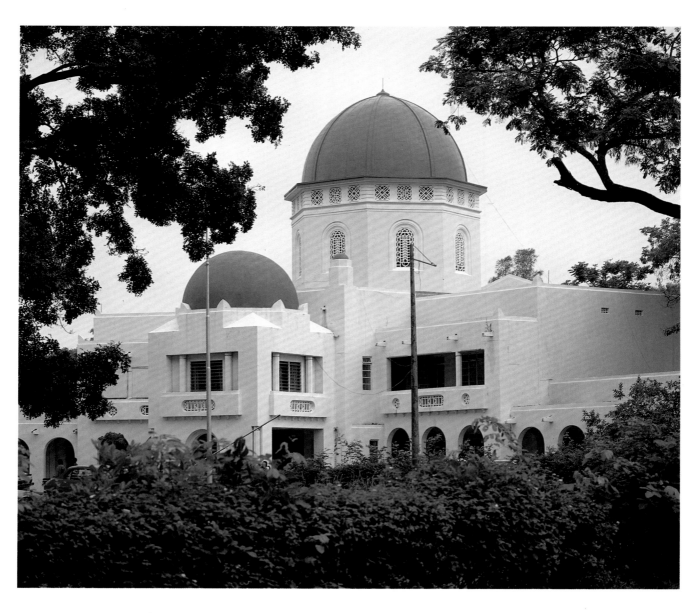

above: Lugard Hall, the old house of assembly in Kaduna

opposite: Kano Central Mosque at sunset

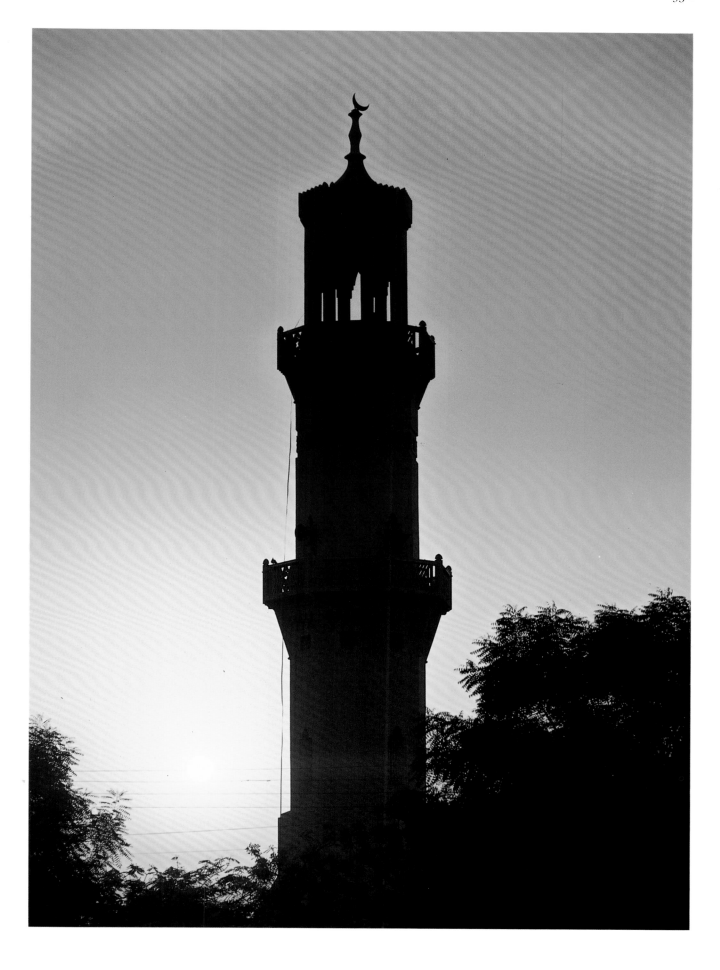

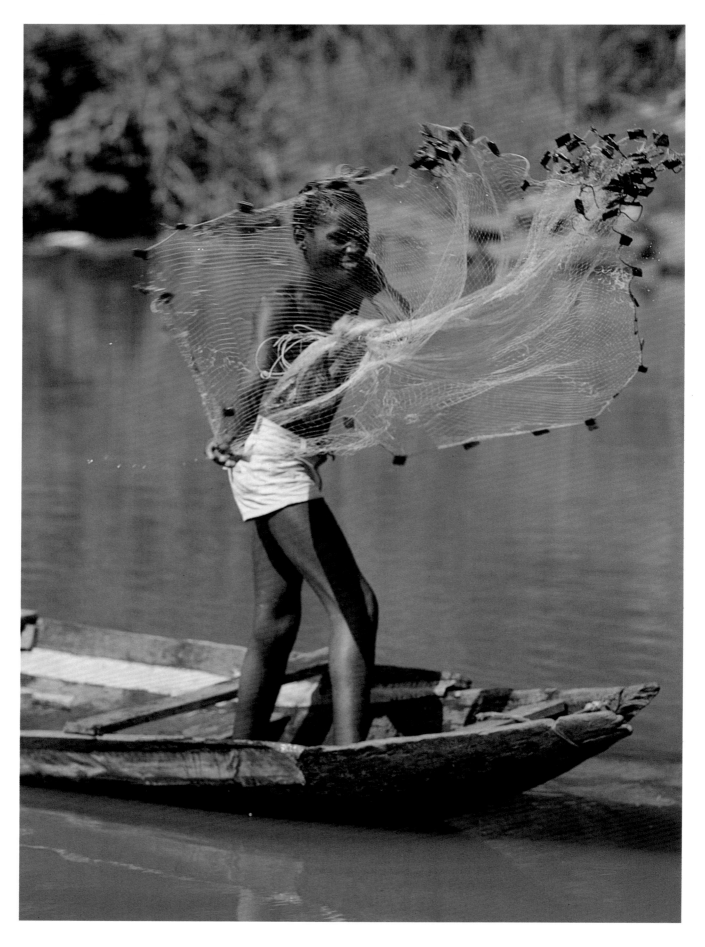

Fishing in Ogbe-Ijoh, Bendel State

in all areas of operations.

Another example has been Ogbe-Ijoh fish farm in Bendel State. It consists of 17 hectares of swamp land, 18 fish ponds, a fish hatchery and a warehouse with equipment. This was designed as an experimental and research centre for fish cultivation in the mangrove swamp and has proved quite successful in providing technical training for fish farmers and as a source of fingerlings to stock their farms. Steps are currently being taken to enhance further this scheme to boost production and increase the number of fish farmers benefiting from the programme.

A rural cassava processing scheme has been initiated aimed at boosting gari production by providing rural centres with dedicated machinery for the use of village communities to process their cassava harvest. Other projects begun in the 70s and still in operation today involve yam, pineapple, palm oil and plantain.

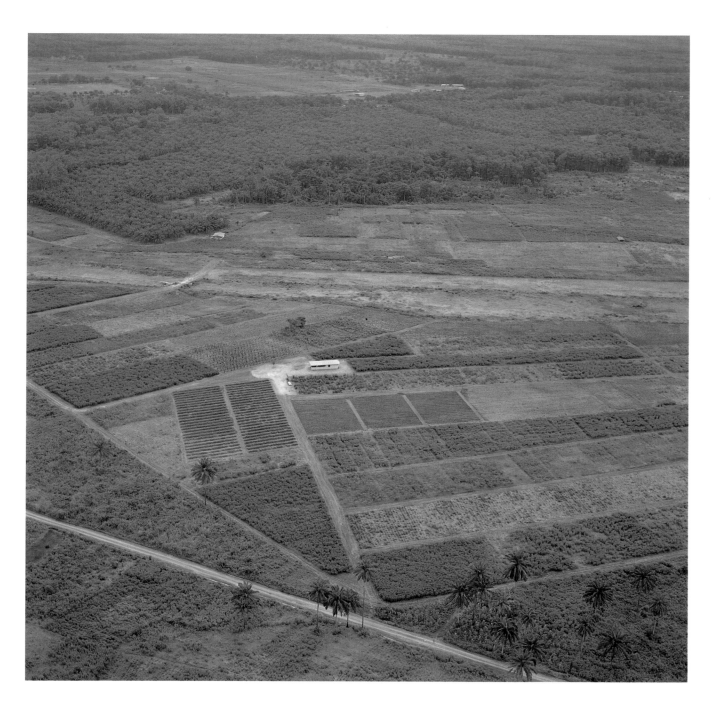

Agbarho Farm Community Development Project, Bendel State

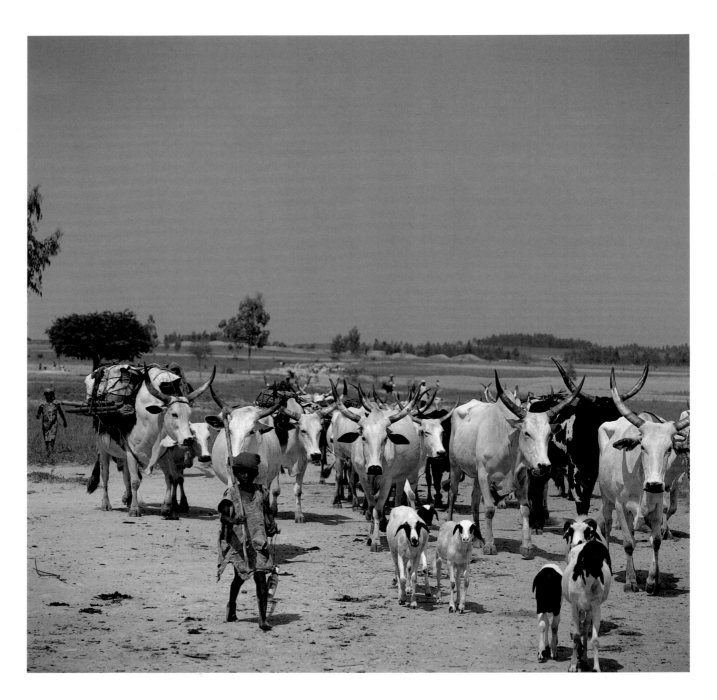

Young Fulani herders with cattle, Plateau State

TRADE, TRANSPORT AND INDUSTRY

FROM the earliest times the various cultural groups in Nigeria had exchanges and contacts with each other. Apart from the importance of the trans-Saharan trade which linked the northern areas with the lands of North Africa, there still exist the extensive oral traditions which recount the growth and spread of the numerous groupings in the main areas. The impression is that the major movements of people and trade were in a north-south direction, but this although in essence true is a simplification of what happened. The size of the country and the various groups emphasised the importance of the great trade arteries. The main artery to the south of the desert area was the Niger-Benue river system which was the means of uniting separate groups by facilitating commercial exchanges. It was the control of these routes and the concomitant revenues that were frequently the subject of political and military disputes. Particularly in the 18th and 19th centuries the arrival of the Europeans in the south reinforced the existing trade systems, bringing new goods and expansion.

The internal 19th century history of Nigeria, especially in the south, is one of great complexity which is complicated further by the presence of Europeans, as traders, explorers and missionaries, in a process which led to the incorporation of the area into the British Empire. The equilibrium of the native societies faced its own internal difficulties whilst the outsider added a new dimension which upset the balance and gave the newcomers the controlling influence.

In the eastern part of the Delta the presence of British traders in the Oil Rivers was supplemented by the arrival of missionaries, initially from Calabar. The Igbo hinterland was penetrated from about 1830 onwards. The need for the regularisation of British mercantile interests saw the establishment of consuls in the area, which along with the presence of naval officers, was merged in due course into a colonial administration. The control of the region was to stop the slave trade, to develop local production of palm oil in particular and to facilitate missionary endeavours. Within a local situation of great turmoil with changes in the economic balance, there were many local power struggles. The situation was regularised with the establishment of a protectorate over the Eastern Delta in 1885 and in the following year the various British companies trading about the Niger came together to form the Royal Niger Company which received its royal charter in that year.

In the Western Delta the old kingdom of Benin was affected by the abolition of the slave trade. It also faced competition from other markets locally in other commodities. These economic difficulties were exacerbated by internal political disputes which culminated in the sack of Benin City in 1897. The other major force in the area, the Aboh kingdom, along with the Itsekiri, faced a similar series of problems. Its once powerful trading base went into decline and was influenced by European traders and explorers. Due to the threat of French interests the economic lifelines of the kingdom were cut off by the Royal Niger Company.

In the southwest the numerous factions of the Yoruba peoples were constantly at war during the 19th century. There was also a great movement of peoples, especially from the open grasslands of north Yorubaland to the subtropical southern forests. The general confused situation was made worse by the influx of traders and the movement of freed slaves into the Lagos area. The state of flux meant there were many local experiments in governmental systems, with the noted emergence of the warrior chief, which

entailed for many the loss of personal freedoms, for protection. The situation required the expansion of the agricultural base. The British came to control the Lagos area from about 1820 where they were concerned to eradicate the slave trade and played host to numerous missionaries. From 1861 the British established their own administration in Lagos, which henceforth was a factor in the politics of the area. Thus Lagos came to be concerned with events in areas such as Ibadan, or came to be a peacemaker among the fighting factions of the Yoruba, as various treaties, for example in 1886 or 1893, demonstrate. In due course British control extended over the whole of the region, to supplement the Colony and Protectorate of Lagos.

below: Roadside cassava stall in Kwara State

opposite: Onitsha market, Anambra State

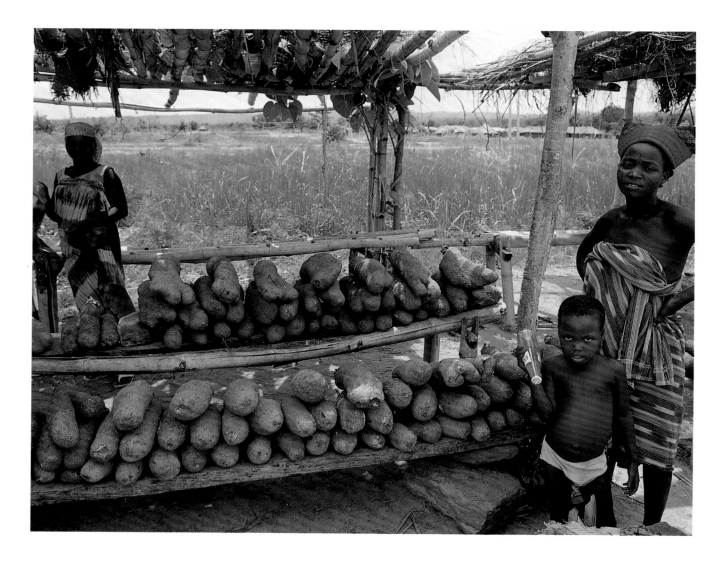

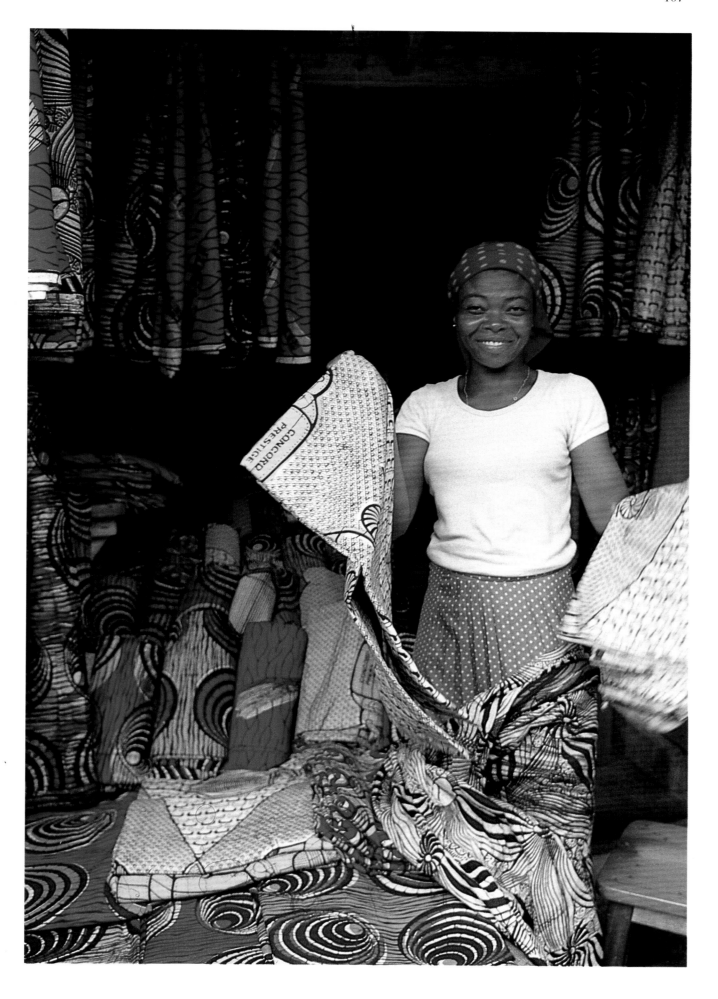

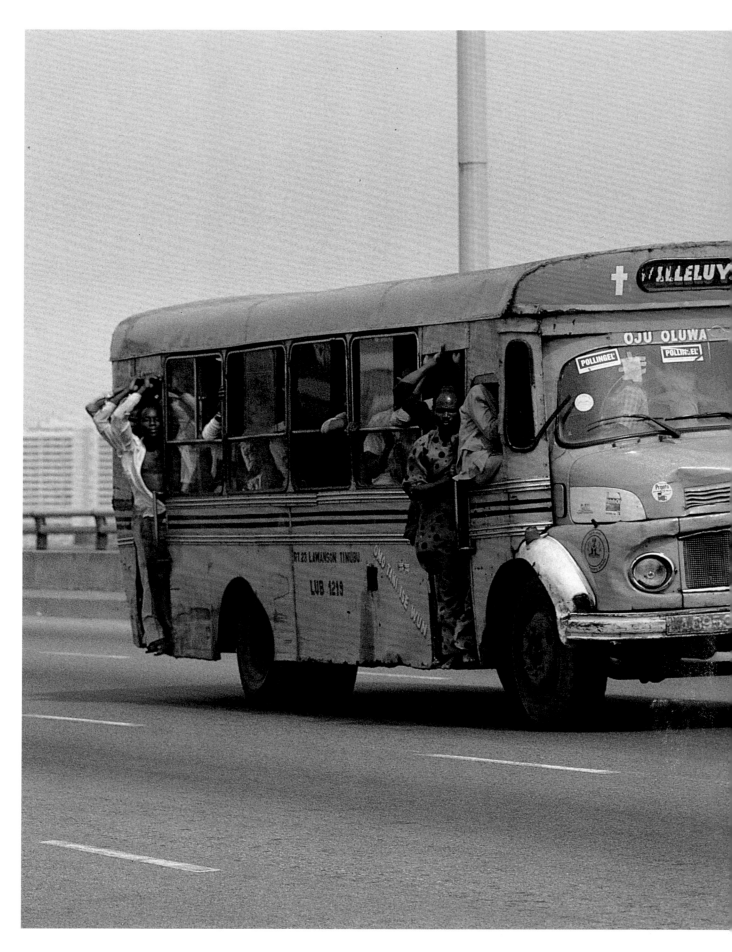

Molue – **Lagos buses**

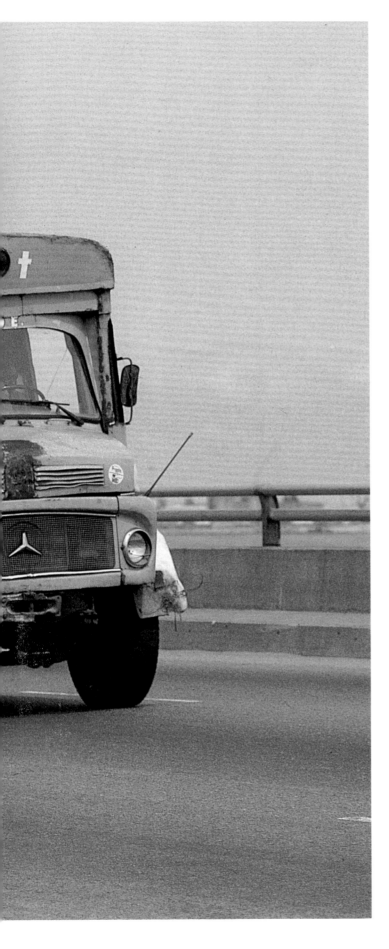

The introduction of banks to expedite financial transactions and the affairs of trade was a major step forward in the 20th century along with the introduction of marketing boards which were designed to fix the prices of produce and to stimulate research, notably in the areas of cocoa, groundnuts, palm oil and cotton. They thus played a very important role in the lives of most Nigerian farmers. The National Bank was established in 1934 as the first indigenous commercial bank in Nigeria.

The period from 1894 up until the end of the First World War was something of a golden age for Nigerian trade in agricultural products. Many local farmers enjoyed a new-found prosperity, with increasing production, high employment, and low taxation. However, after 1918 the general depression which affected world markets had its repercussions within Nigeria, and despite the brief upturn in the mid-1920s, this situation was to persist through the 30s till the end of the Second World War. During the 1950s trade in a variety of goods, most notably agricultural, participated in the post-war boom and a level of prosperity began to return to the country. The early years of the 1960s saw significant trade agreements with Japan (1962) and the Soviet Union (1963). Nigeria hosted its first International Trade Fair in 1962. Other landmarks in the progress of the now independent nation included the inauguration of new currency denominations in 1965, airport developments in 1963 and a host of other industrial projects.

During the 1960s Nigeria was able to achieve some major economic developments. A significant factor was the spread of television and radio services, with a new Nigerian Television Service building constructed in 1963. A major programme saw moves to industrialisation, whilst some traditional agricultural crops, such as cocoa and rubber, were expanded. The growing nation also required an effective transport infrastructure which led to the development of roads, railways, ports and airways. As aspirations changed there was an acceleration of the process of a move to urban areas from the countryside.

—110—

The oil-boom and trade in the products of energy marked the decade of the 1970s and succeeded in establishing Nigerian economic prosperity. Wealth derived from oil production has, for example, been responsible for funding the construction of the new capital in the central Federal Territory at Abuja, and in previous years the impressive infrastructures in Lagos as well as roads, bridges, and industrial and agricultural schemes throughout the country.

However, the fluctuations within the world oil markets and the depression of prices in the 1980s brought about a change in direction of the economy. The economic difficulties that the country began to experience were compounded by international events over which Nigeria had

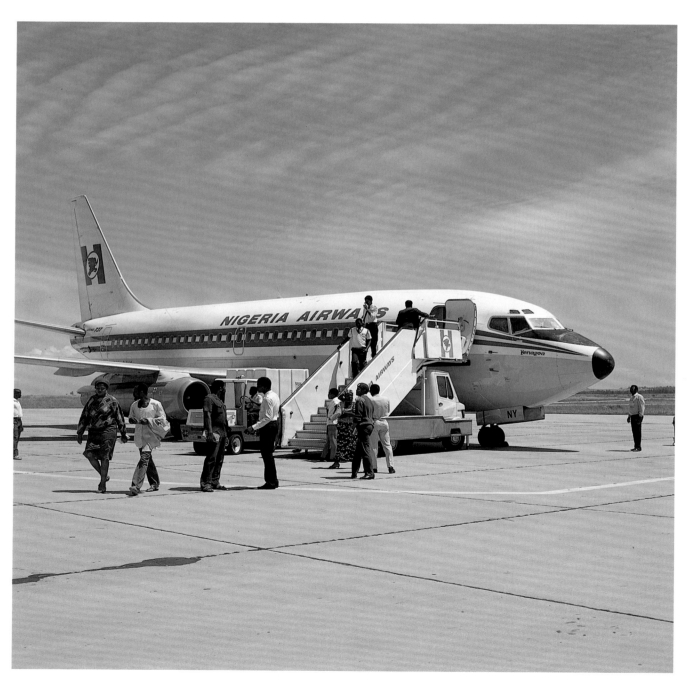

Nigerian Airways Boeing 737 at Jos Airport, Plateau State

no control. The new sense of reality and determination now present within the country is witnessing the maintenance and expansion of certain sectors of the economy, especially in regard to energy resources. The gas and petrochemical resources of the country are impressive. In the petroleum sphere, oil exports still provide Nigeria's main source of foreign currency earnings.

As the decade of the 1980s draws to a close Nigeria will consider its many achievements in the recent past and can be confident in the future. The land has vast natural resources which its people have the talent and imagination to develop fruitfully. Armed with resources, experience and confidence its future is destined to confirm it as 'the Giant of Africa'.

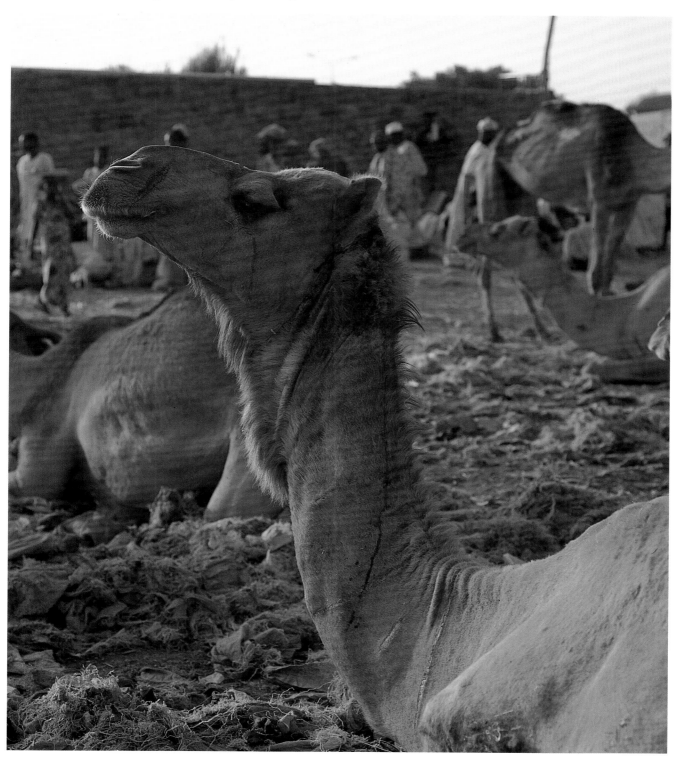

Kano camel market

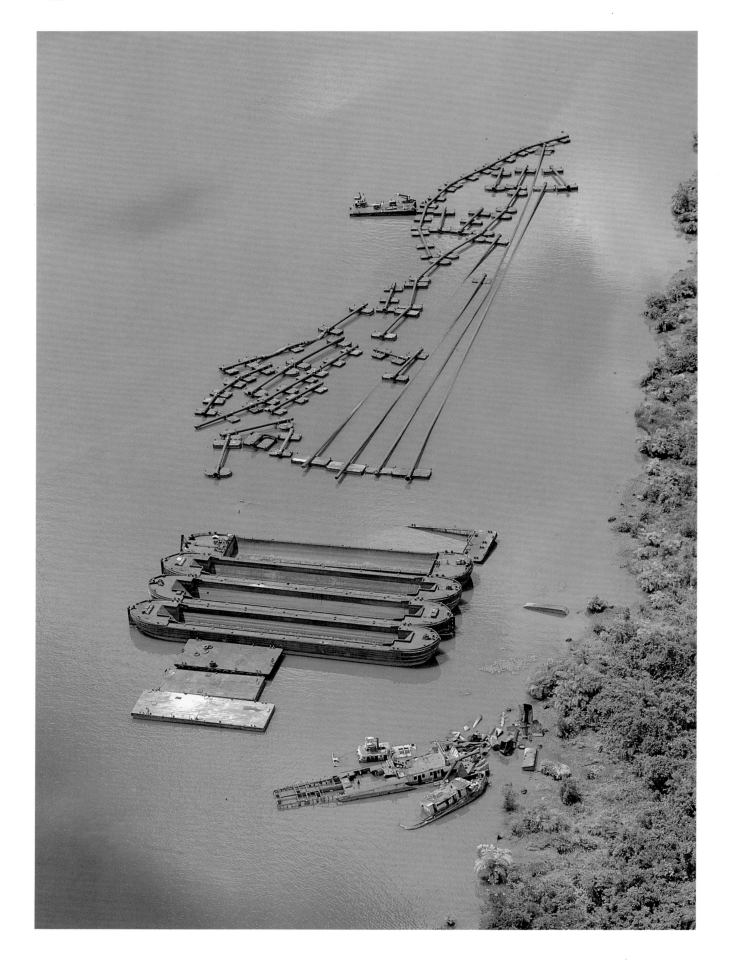

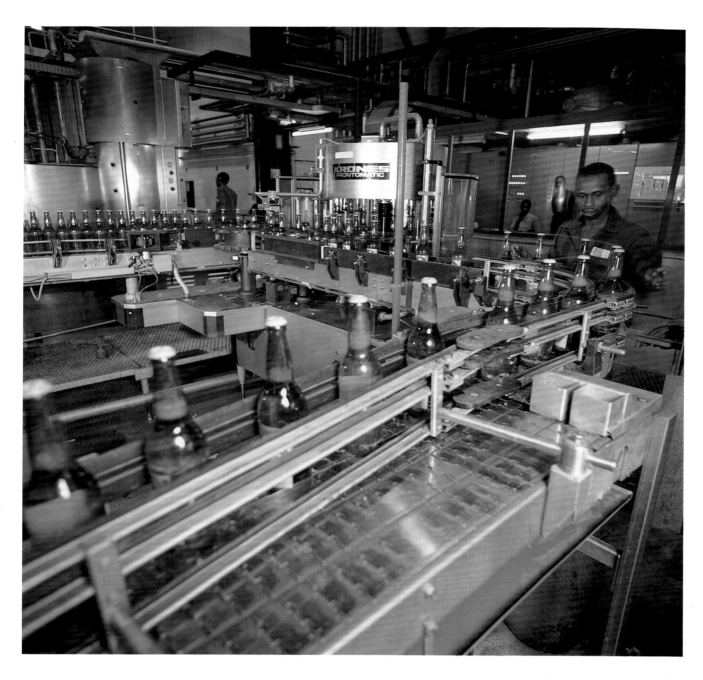

above: A filling line in the Pabod brewery, Port Harcourt, Rivers State

opposite: Barges on the river, Warri, Bendel State

—114—

TRANSPORT

Until the end of the 19th century transportation by head porterage, donkeys, camels and, above all, heavy barges and canoes on the extensive waterways had served the Nigerian population's needs. However, the increasing industrialisation and agricultural production within the country demanded that methods of transportation also be improved. Railways were therefore built to replace the traditional forms of transport. In 1895 the first line was begun from Lagos to Kano, succeeded by the line from Port Harcourt to the north. After the advent of the motor car and the improvement in road transport, the construction of railways was also accompanied by a corresponding upsurge in the construction of new roads. Lorries began to challenge the dominance of

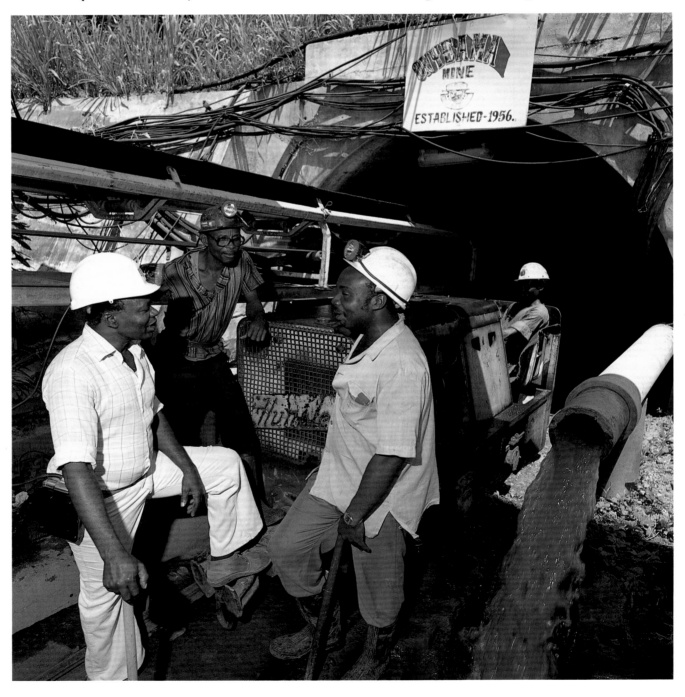

Miners at the Onyeama coal mine in Enugu, Anambra State

the rail system. They had the advantage of more flexible mobility once roads had been created for them and also travelled East to West whereas rail building had been restricted by the lines from North to South imposed mostly by the demands of the export trade.

The advances in the methods of communication, as well as the extension of the industrial and agricultural base, obviously wrought great changes in other aspects of the environment. Many towns and regions declined in importance whilst others grew. Borno, for instance, in the north-east, which had previously been an area of great political and cultural significance, occasioned by its position at the end of the trans-Saharan trade route, was replaced by Kano, whose rise under the Sokoto Caliphate had now been accelerated by its position as a railway centre controlling communications to the south. Similarly, many new settlements grew up along the new roads and railway links. Port Harcourt, where new shipping facilities had been constructed, increased in importance because of export demands.

The construction of railways in the country began when the need arose to find a means of moving produce from the hinterland to the coast for export. Railways in Nigeria were then operated and managed as a government department until October 1955, when the Nigerian Railway Corporation was established as a public corporation.

With the exception of Akwa-Ibom, Bendel, Cross Rivers, Gongola and Ondo States, all other States of the Federation are served by the existing 1,607 millimetre gauge single-track system. The rail lines, covering a total of 3,505 kilometres, consist of two routes linking the two main ocean ports of Lagos and Port Harcourt with industrial and commercial centres in the country. These routes converge in Kaduna and then branch off to the north-east and north-west, terminating respectively at Nguru in Borno State and Kaura Namoda in Sokoto State.

Nigerian Railways provides local and commuter passenger services as well as carrying goods; its major freight consists of groundnuts, groundnut oil, groundnut cake, palm produce, cement and salt. Others are columbite, petroleum products, hides and skins.

Until 1959, when Nigeria Airways was created, domestic air operations were handled by the West African Airways Corporation (WAAC). Although a few private airlines (owned by Nigerians) have now joined in the provision of domestic air services, Nigeria Airways still dominates the domestic scene. The Airways company now also runs scheduled flights to some major cities of the world, competing in this regard with other well-known international airlines. Within the country, the Lagos, Port Harcourt and Kano airports have been developed to full international standards, while those in Calabar, Sokoto and Maiduguri have also been equipped to meet many of the requirements of international air transport. Apart from these, however, almost all state capitals have airports for domestic air travel and airfreight of goods from port to port.

INDUSTRY

Before the colonial period a number of traditional industries existed. Chief amongst these were saltmaking and metalworking. Much of Northern Nigeria's salt was obtained through the trans-Saharan route and derived from Saharan sources. However, in the north-east another centre had been established around Lake Chad, which also supplied the invaluable product of natron, or potash. The peoples in the Benue basin mostly derived their salt from Awe in Adamawa, while the Nembe and Itsekiri areas provided most of the salt demands in the south of the country.

Iron and tin ore were mined around the Bauchi Plateau and Mandaran Hills and from there traded all over Nigeria. Although the ore originated from these areas, the inhabitants of other regions were involved in the production of metal goods. Much fine smithy work, for example, was done in Hausaland to the north. Domestic ore production and metalworking still continued to be effective after 1900 although under increasing pressure from European imports. Tin mining reached a level of importance with the status of a modern industry in the early 20th century but it never fully recovered from the commercial effects of the First World War and suffered especially in the early 1930s.

The reserves of tin found on Jos Plateau and Udi Hill were natural resources which were exploited during the 20th century. Ore smelting had long been one of Nigeria's indigenous technologies, but the nature of the industry changed dramatically in the 20th century.

As in all spheres of trade, industrial development was severely affected by the post-World War depression and did not regain momentum until the 1950s when large enterprises like UAC switched more of their investment to manufacturing and the energy industry began to develop. Through various financial incentives the Government encouraged the establishment of manufacturing industry to offset the cost of imports. Throughout this period new factories continued to spring up in Port Harcourt, Lagos, Ibadan and Kaduna, in industries such as cement, brewing, textiles, ceramics and furniture.

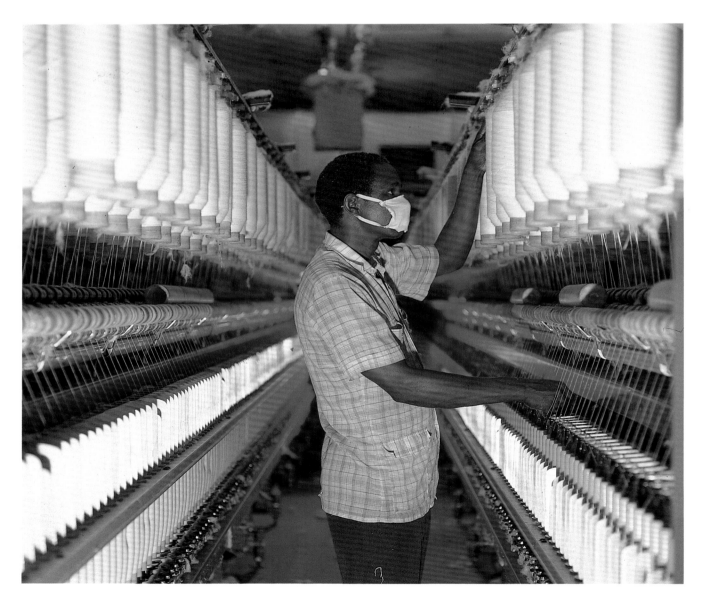

Ring spinning in the Aba Textile Mills, Rivers State

Regional specialisation within industry was becoming more readily apparent, and this concentration of interconnecting services and manufacturing, coupled with the resultant regional pools of skilled labour and the application of new technology, contributed a great step forward in industrial productivity.

A number of cement factories were established in various parts of the country, located to take advantage of large deposits of limestone, for example, those at Ewekoro, Shagamu and Nkalagu.

The iron and steel plants located in Aladja constitute part of another major industry established in Nigeria in recent years. An integrated iron and steel plant at Ajaokuta is also under construction.

Four major vehicle assembly plants were built for the production of passenger and commercial vehicles in the country, the most important of which are the Peugeot plant at Kaduna and the Volkswagen plant in Lagos. Other industries for the production of consumer goods such as milk, sugar, soaps, bicycles and various types of tyres have also been established to cater for domestic demands.

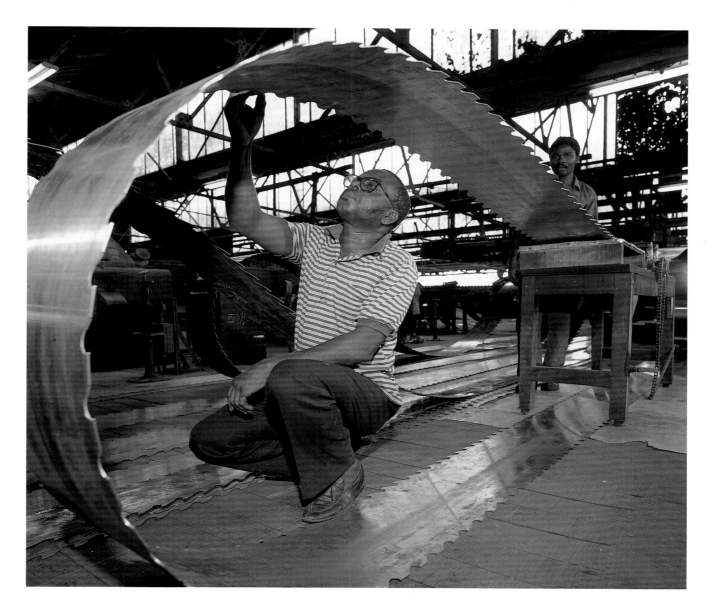

Checking a band-saw at African Timber and Plywood (ATP) in Sapele, Bendel State

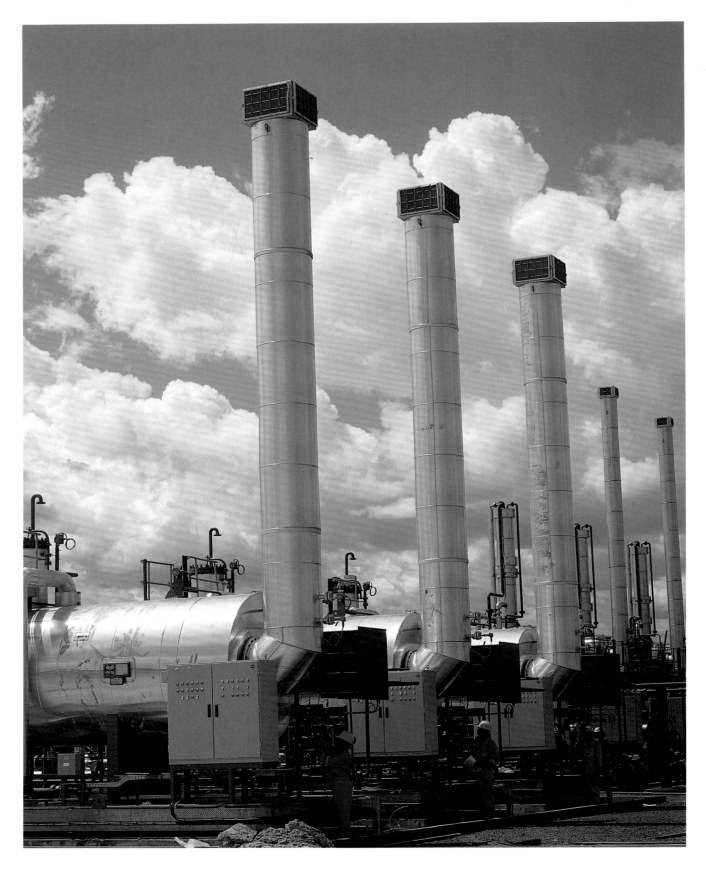

Part of the Utorogu gas plant near Warri

Delta Steel Plant in Warri, Bendel State

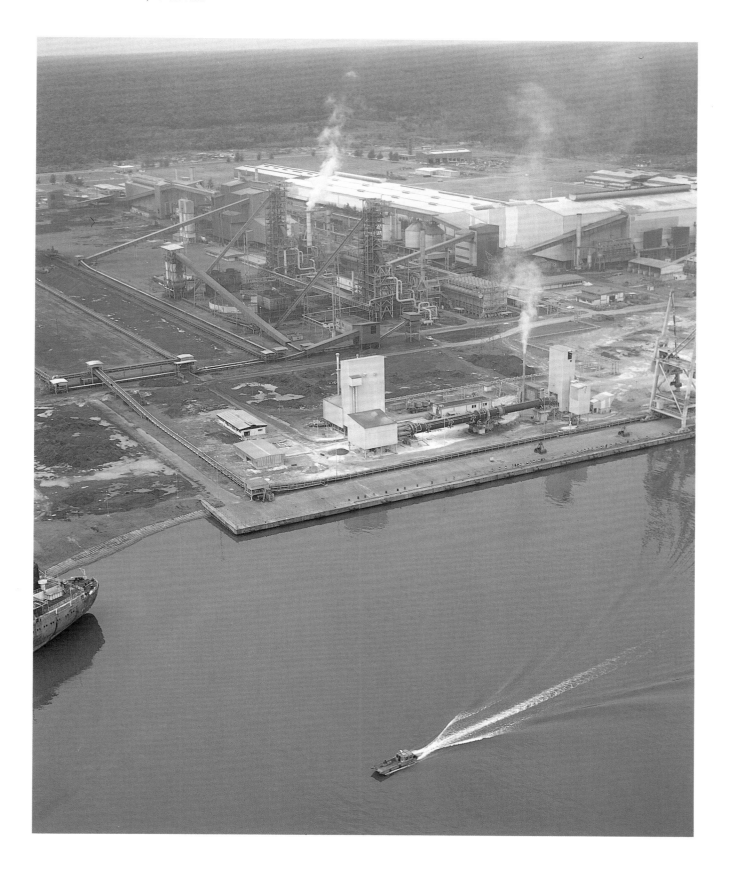

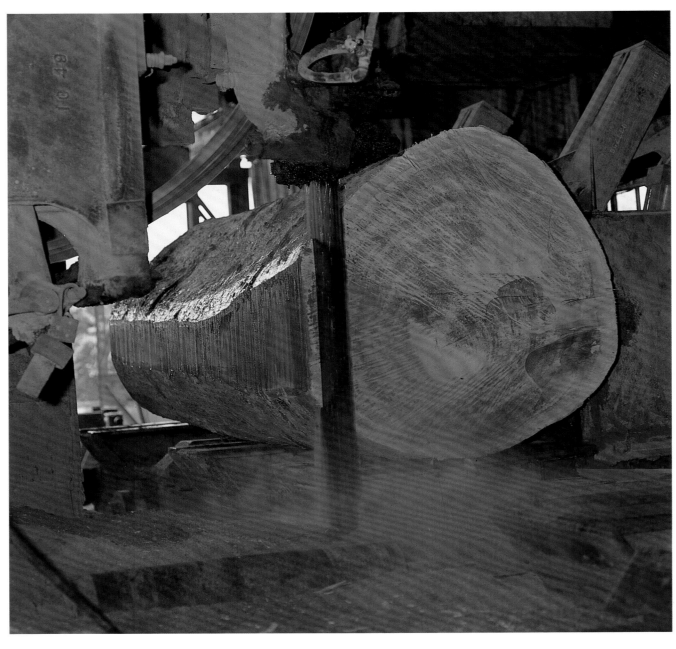

**Work in progress at African Timber and Plywood (ATP) in Sapele,
Bendel State**

ENERGY AND OIL

THE rapid development of the oil industry in the 1960s is probably the single most important factor in Nigeria's economic development. The product which was to transfigure the whole economy of Nigeria was first systematically investigated in 1938 by Shell D'Arcy. Shell's first base was established at Owerri and despite previous negative indications as to the existence of oil anywhere in West Africa, the company persisted with its seismic and exploration programme. The area of operation initially included the whole of Nigeria but eventually the search focused on the Niger Delta. Enormous funds were expended with no visible reward and the project nearly came to a disappointing end before the discovery which was to make such a vital impact on Nigeria's recent history. Nigerian oil proved at first very difficult to locate. It was present in relatively small accumulations which were scattered in different terrains, mostly in difficult, inaccessible areas. However, when viewed in total, the reserves were to prove of enormous extent.

The 1950s was the decade of major petroleum discoveries. From modest beginnings in the 1950s oil production accelerated rapidly in the 1960s. The increased demand for oil was a great boost for the whole Nigerian economy at a time when its traditional cash crop income was decreasing due to a fall in world market prices.

The series of breakthroughs in Nigeria's oil production began significantly in 1953 when Shell's Akata-1 well produced quantities of oil, but unfortunately not of sufficient size to justify commercial production. However, 1956 saw the discovery at Oloibiri in Rivers State which did at last prove commercially viable. Later in the same year more oil was found at Afam, also in Rivers State. Then began the construction of pipelines from Oloibiri to Port Harcourt to facilitate export. The first cargo of crude oil was exported on 17 February 1958. An average of approximately 4,400 barrels per day were being produced by the end of that year.

As the search for oil intensified during 1958 and 1959, other companies decided to join in the exploration. More discoveries were made by Shell at Ebubu and Bomu in Rivers State and Ughelli in Bendel State. Already these discoveries and their potential had transformed Nigeria into one of the key oil producing countries in the world. After its small initial success, increased scientific expertise allowed Shell to locate and develop further oil fields in the 1960s and 1970s, with computer-aided techniques becoming an essential feature of present-day operations. Following the rapid increase in production at Oloibiri and other new fields, Shell decided to move its headquarters to Port Harcourt where harbour facilities and communications networks were more suitable for the direction of oil export. The company set up offices, training bases, workshops and residential areas to aid its operations.

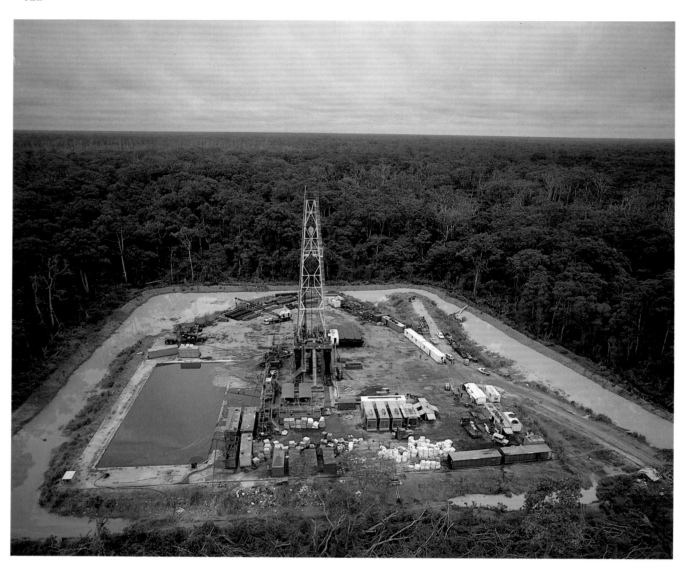

above: Saipem rig drilling at Okwuibome in Bendel State

opposite: Proposed site for the Finima LNG plant in Rivers State

As the level of production rose it was also found necessary to build a suitable oil terminal at Bonny. The harbour bar at Bonny, however, severely restricted the draught of shipping. A dredging programme was therefore instigated in 1959. The bar was initially dredged to 8.2 metres then to 11.3; from 1961 Bonny terminal was in operation, with initially four tanks and 30,000 barrels capacity. Production immediately exceeded 50,000 and the company fulfilled an obligation to the Government to build a refinery in Nigeria; this was the Alesa-Eleme refinery, which was originally owned and financed by Shell-BP. Today this and the other refineries at Warri and Kaduna are fully owned and run by the Nigerian National Petroleum Corporation. In 1962 under the terms of the concession, Shell relinquished half of its acreage holding, and this in turn attracted other international companies. There were 14 companies in total in 1970, including Gulf, Texaco, Mobil, Elf and Agip, at which time offshore areas of the Niger Delta were opened up for exploration. Oil was now a major industry, employing over 3,000 people directly, with some 500,000 barrels a day being produced by 1967, thus creating considerable revenue for the country. The Civil War caused great disruption around Port Harcourt and production was in fact suspended from August 1967 to September 1968. At the end of the crisis the oil company returned to Bonny and Port Harcourt, where the reconstruction and rehabilitation of the facilities were completed in record time. Before the War the fields in the Western

Division of the company's operations were connected with Bonny by the Trans-Niger pipeline. This work was completed by 1965, but the increasing quantity of oil in Bendel State and the introduction of very large tankers required the construction of a new terminal at Forcados and a 93 kilometre pipeline to connect it to the producing fields. The pipeline was completed in 1969 and the Forcados terminal commissioned in 1971; by 1970 production was reaching 1,000,000 barrels a day.

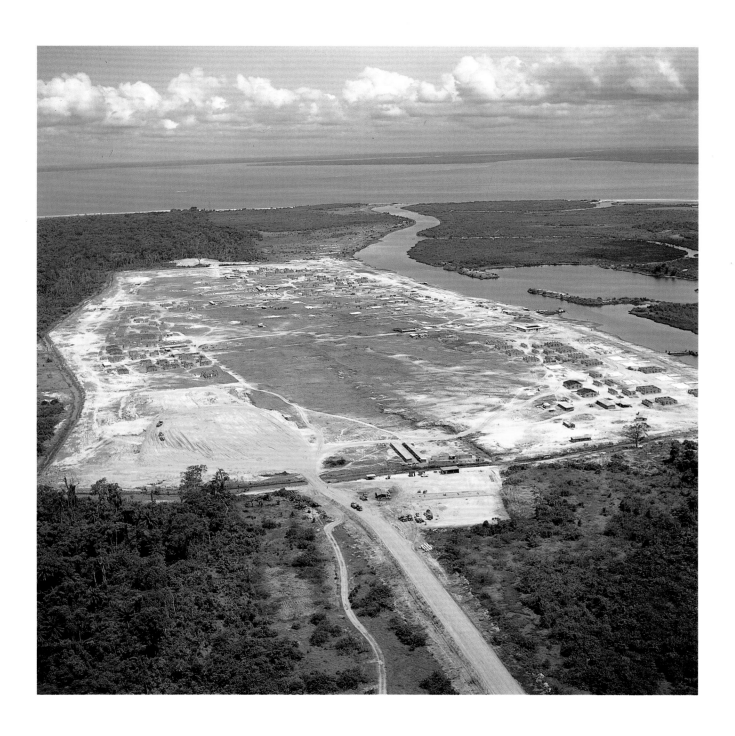

A considerable number of exploration and appraisal/development wells were drilled in the 1960s, totalling more than 70 per annum from 1964-69, with over 110 in 1966. By 1970 the oil industry was responsible for about 95% of the nation's foreign exchange earnings, of which Shell was the major contributor. Shell had produced 289 million barrels of oil since 1958, and had drilled 866 wells with 32 production fields.

The Nigerian oil industry, like the international industry, was subject to various changes during the 1970s. In 1971 the price per barrel was $2 in the world market. By 1974, after the first world oil price increase,

Nigeria was producing 2.2 million barrels per day and Shell's share of this production had risen to 1.4 million. This represented the highest point of the country's total oil output. Production remained more or less at this level, despite economies in consumption by the Western industrialised nations during the mid-1970s, until 1980 when the second world oil price increase led to a huge fall in demand. New refineries were opened at Warri in 1978 and Kaduna in 1980 to bring production to 260,000 barrels per day. In line with OPEC agreements, the price per barrel had now risen to around $35, but with the international demand so low this price

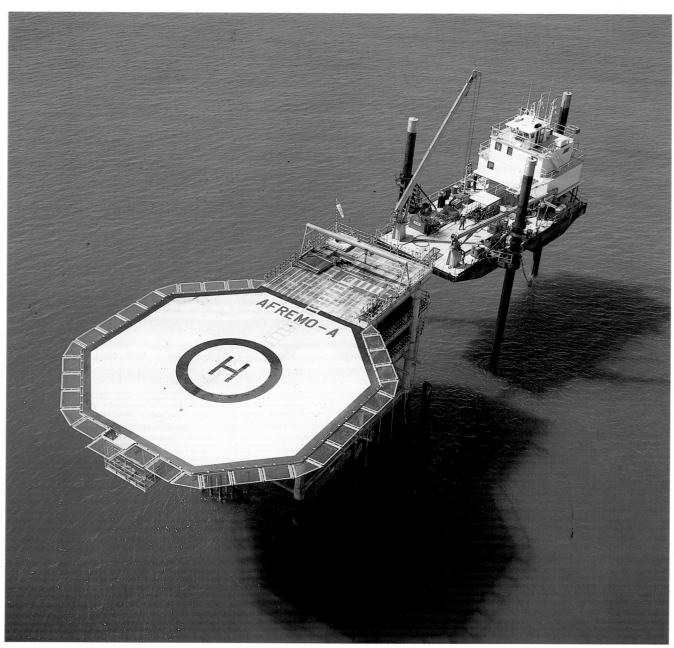

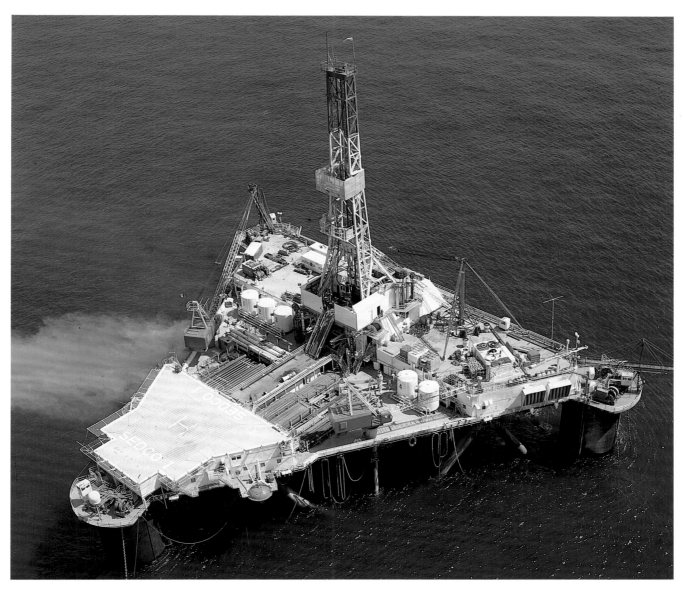

opposite: **Afremo platform, an offshore installation of Shell's Western Division**

above: **Sedco 1 drilling rig**

could not be sustained. Later in the 1980s prices and production levels were to drop dramatically.

By 1980 the government's revenues from oil amounted to approximately $23 billion, but was destined to fall to a quarter of that in the next six years.

Shell's Forcados and Bonny terminals have a combined storage capacity of over 13 million barrels. Loading rates of 6,500 tonnes/hour and 11,000 tonnes/hour can be achieved at Bonny and Forcados respectively. The two single buoy moorings at each terminal lie 25 km offshore. They are each capable of handling up to 320,000 tonne tankers deadweight; Bonny also has three inshore buoy moorings for tankers of 18,000-135,000 tonnes. The length of pipelines now extend over 5,600 kms. Shell Nigeria has 83 producing oil fields and 8 main trunk lines. With the administrative headquarters in Lagos, the company operates through two divisions: the Eastern Division based at Port Harcourt, and the Western Division at Warri. The total staff of the company in Nigeria in 1988 is some 5,000 staff, of which about 3% are ex-patriates.

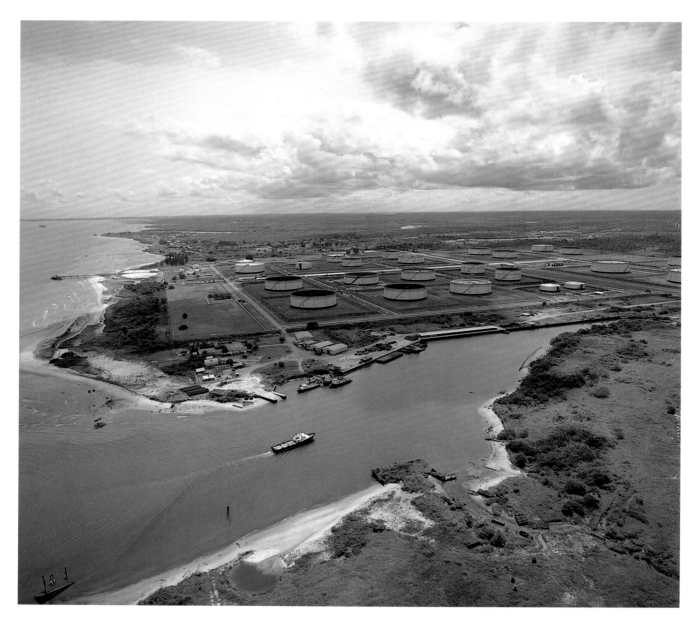

Shell's interest in efficient production has for a long time encouraged its development of manpower training schemes, adding to the educational opportunities available within the country. These include on the job training for those employed in immediate work in the industry, more advanced technical training, taking place mostly at Port Harcourt and Warri, general development training with its centre in Warri, and a high number of scholarships, mostly in Nigerian institutes of education. In addition, many employees have been posted on overseas assignment, where they occupy responsible positions in various Shell operating companies located in other countries. The total Shell budget on training over the last five years amounted to almost 25 million naira.

above: The Bonny Oil Terminal, south of Port Harcourt

opposite: Utorogu gas plant near Warri

Gas has also been an important by-product of oil exploration and production. Vast gas fields have been discovered which should have far-reaching consequences for the future Nigerian economy. Some gas has been supplied for many years to industries and power stations in the Niger Delta. More recent developments in the 1980s – with natural gas liquids (NGL) and liquid petroleum gas (LPG) in which Nigeria is very rich – have indicated that gas will now come to the forefront of energy development. Major plants have been constructed at Alakiri and Utorogu to supply quality gas for the manufacture of fertilizer at Onne and power generation near Lagos. The liquid natural gas (LNG) project planned for Bonny will be

able to export some 4 million tonnes of LNG to Europe from 1995. This project between the Nigerian National Petroleum Corporation, Shell, Agip and Elf is an important investment in the nation's rich gas reserves and Shell is proud of its role as the technical leader.

Until the discovery of oil, coal was Nigeria's prime source of energy for electricity generation and the fuel for running the nation's fleet of railway locomotives. Coal exists in commercial quantity in Onyeama and Okpara in the Enugu coal fields of Anambra State, and in Owukpa and Okabba in Benue State. Onyeama and Okpara are underground mines while the deposits at Owukpa and Okabba are open-cast. Coking

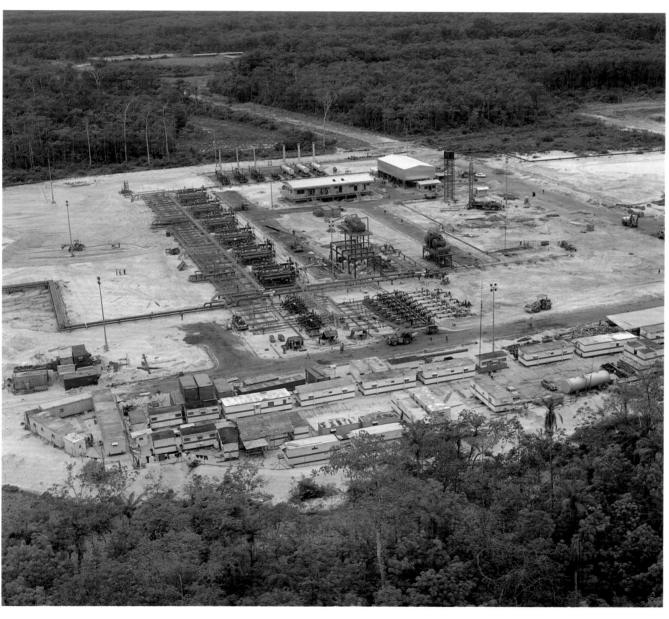

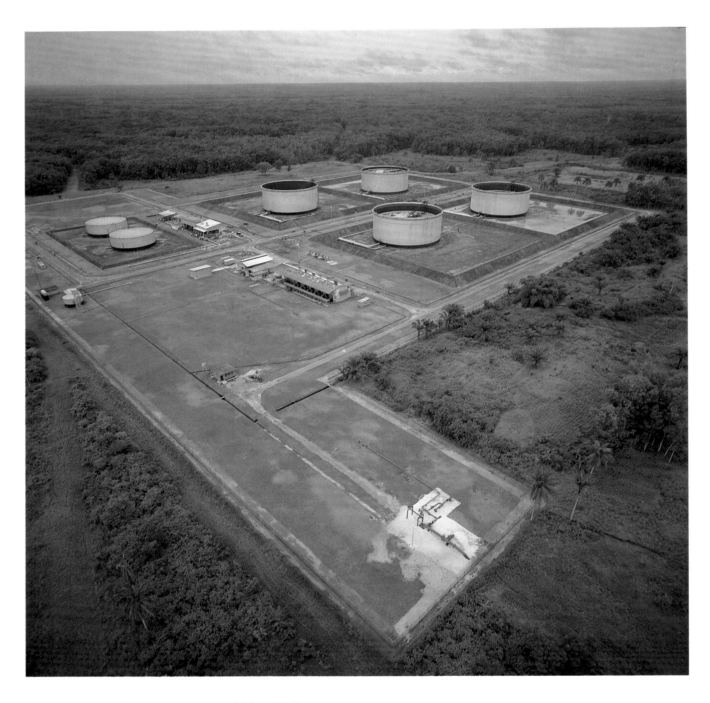

**Ughelli Quality Control Centre, in the Western Division of Shell
Petroleum Development Company**

Shell staff housing in Warri, Bendel State

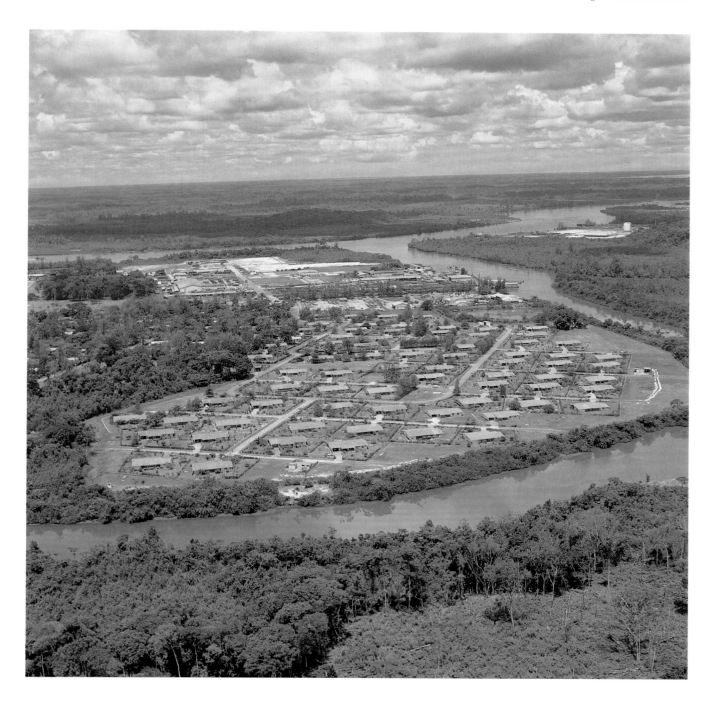

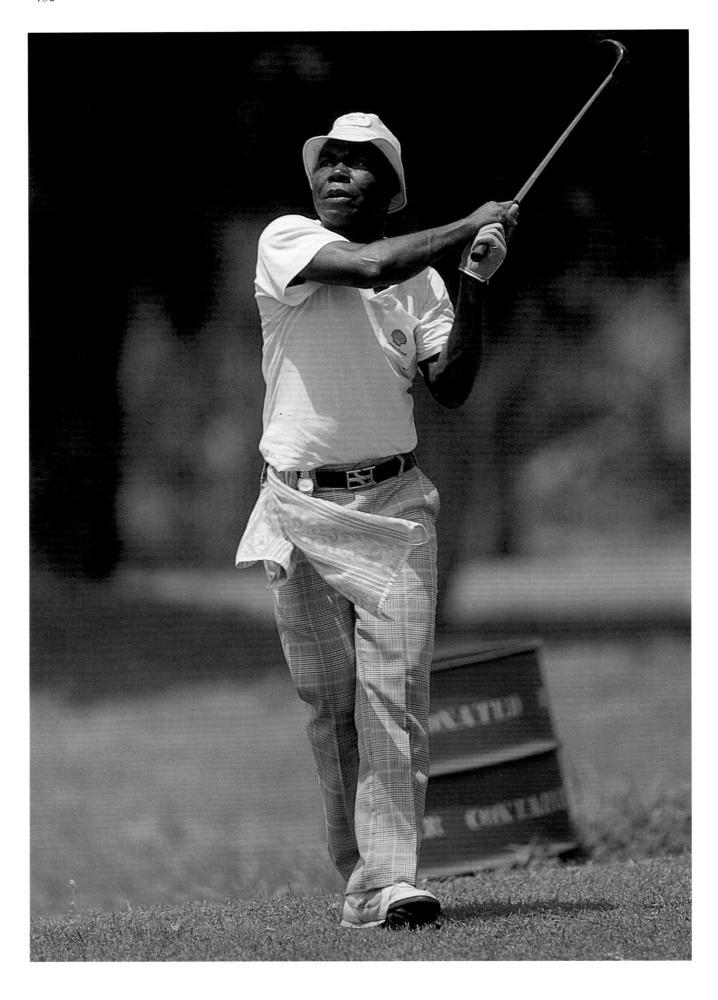

SPORT

SPORT has always been a part of Nigerian culture. The pre-colonial riverine communities of the Niger Delta were famed for their competitive regattas, while wrestling contests were common in village squares all over the country.

British colonial rule encouraged sports competitions, with the Empire Day Games serving as occasions for schools within a district or province to compete for laurels in athletics. Field and track events were the first form of organised sports in the country because they required few specialised facilities.

In April 1947 the first ever All-Nigeria Athletics Championships took place in Ibadan. Its success encouraged the country to inaugurate an international championship between Nigeria and the Gold Coast (now Ghana) later that year. Less than a decade later Nigeria won her first gold medal in the high jump, with Emmanuel Ifeajuna leaping over 6 feet 8 inches at the 1954 Commonwealth Games in Vancouver, Canada.

Again, in 1966, Sam Igun won another gold for the country in the 'three jumps' event at the Commonwealth Games in Kingston, Jamaica. The country's 4 x 100 metres quartet also won the gold at the Commonwealth Games in Brisbane, Australia. Nigeria won further medals in the female events at the Commonwealth Games in Cardiff, in 1966, when Violet Odogwu won the bronze in the long jump. Modupe Oshikoya achieved an outstanding feat when she won a bronze, silver and gold in three different events at the tenth Commonwealth Games in Christchurch, New Zealand. At the Olympic level, the country has produced some of the world's finest athletes, with Chidi Imo and Innocent Egbunike emerging as two of the world's fastest men in their respective track events.

Apart from athletics, boxing was perhaps the one other sport that propelled Nigeria into the limelight in the 1950s. Nojeem Maiyegun won the bronze medal in the middleweight division at the eighteenth Olympic Games in Tokyo, Japan, in 1964, while Isaac Ikhuoria again performed the same feat in the same weight division at the Munich Olympics of 1972. Nigeria won its first silver medal in Olympic boxing, through Peter Konyegwachie, at the 1984 Los Angeles Olympics.

Hogan 'Kid' Bassey emerged as the first Nigerian to win a world title in professional boxing when he became featherweight boxing champion of the world in 1957. He was soon followed in 1962 by Dick Tiger, who not only won the middleweight title in that year but went on to win the light-heavyweight title as well. A third world champion has recently emerged in Bash Ali.

Golf at the Ikoyi Club in Lagos

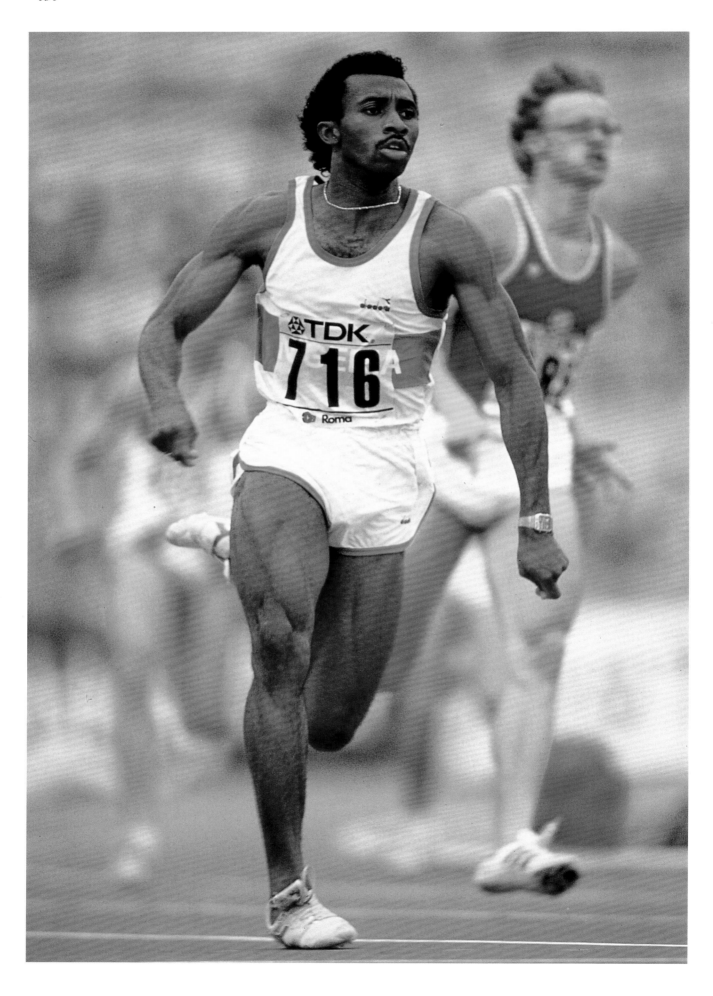

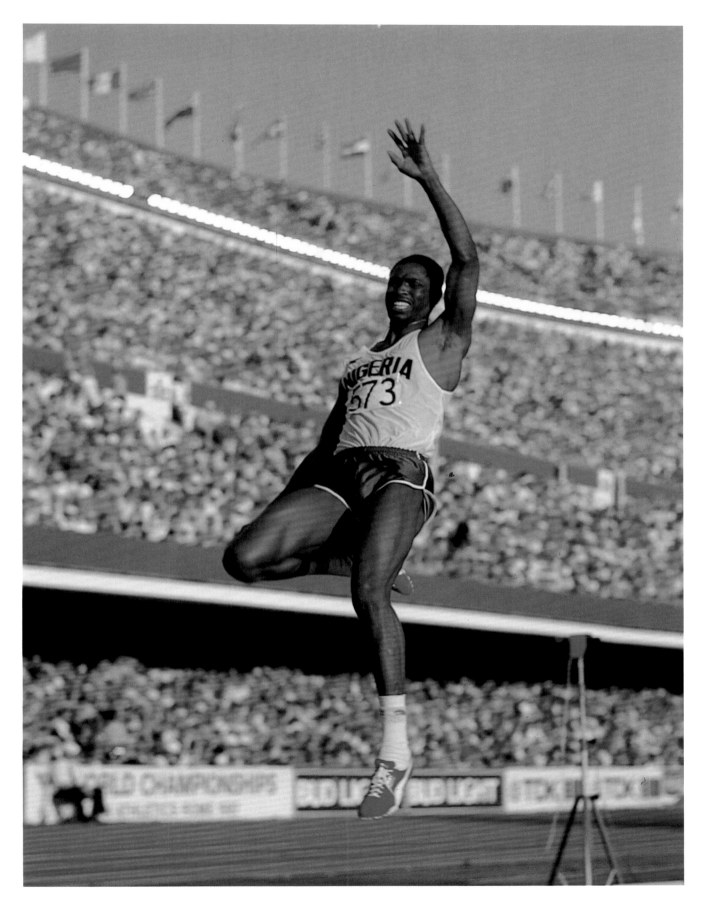

opposite: Innocent Egbunike takes part in the 1987 World Championships in Rome (courtesy All-Sport Photographic Limited)

above: Yussuf Alli competing at the World Championships in 1983 (courtesy All-Sport Photographic Limited)

Perhaps no other game is as popular with Nigerians as football. Although the Nigerian Football Association was formed in 1945, the game did not quite capture the imagination of the people until 1949 when the first Nigerian national side went on a tour of Britain.

Today, Nigerian football has attained world standard, with the nation's under-17 team (The Golden Eaglets) winning the first ever Kodak World Cup in that category, in Beijing, China, in 1984.

Football is almost matched in popularity by table tennis. Nigeria is pre-eminent in Africa at this game and one of its players is a past holder of the Commonwealth men's singles' title. Cricket is also a game in which Nigeria has dominated the West African scene for many years. Lawn tennis and golf so far have a limited appeal but Nduka Odizor is well known in Wimbledon circles whilst some professional golfers have emerged recently to win fame for themselves and the nation.

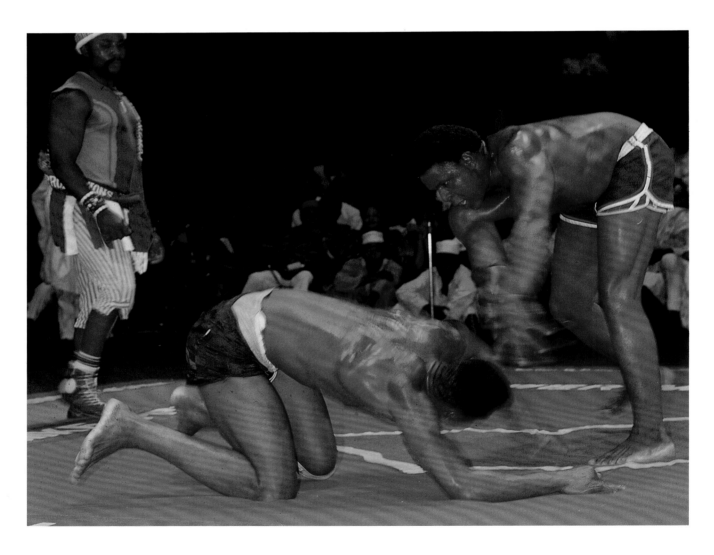

above: Traditional African wrestling at the National Stadium, Lagos

opposite: The Imo State University in Okigwe

EDUCATION AND HEALTH

IN old Nigerian society, education was generally designed as a preparation for adult life and induction into society. It emphasized social responsibility, skill, work and ethics and provided a means of encouraging political participation and teaching of moral values. Children and adolescents learnt through ceremonies, rituals, imitation, recitation and demonstration. They were involved in practical farming, weaving, cooking, carving

and so on, whilst intellectual training comprised the study of local history, legend, riddles, proverbs, and related skills. Education in Nigeria has been influenced significantly by both the Christian and Islamic religions. Islamic religion reached the savannah region of West Africa in the 8th century and spread to the part of Northern Nigeria called Kanem-Bornu region in 1085 AD. It later reached Hausaland in the early 14th century. As Islam spread so did Islamic

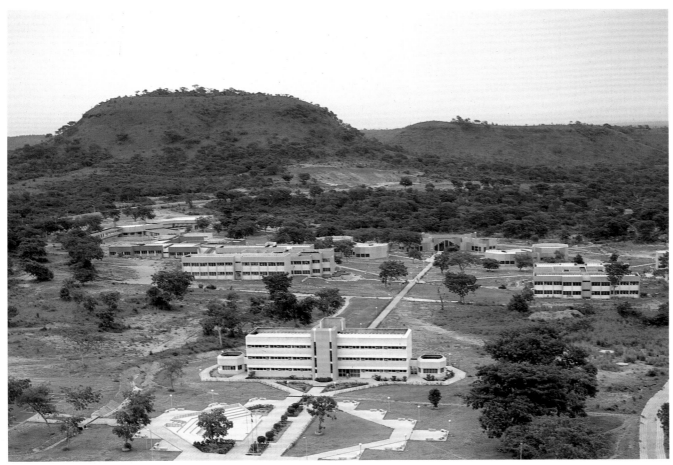

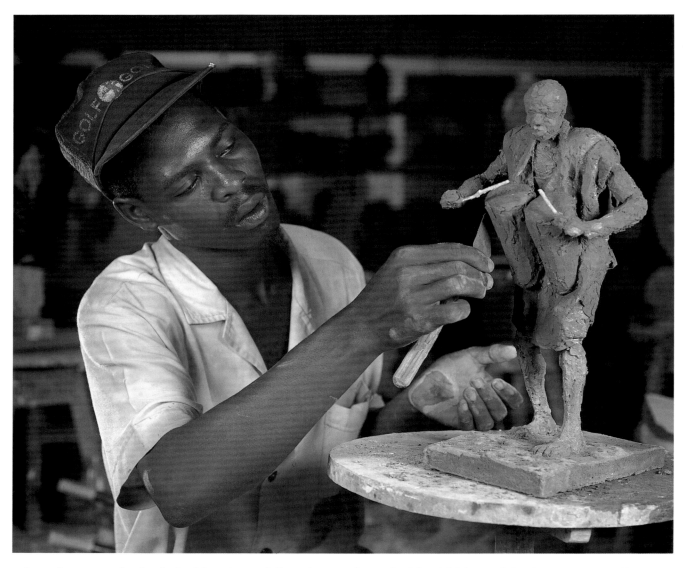

education, particularly in Northern Nigeria and parts of Yorubaland in the later 18th century. While Islam has had its impact on Nigerian education from the 14th century to the present, the great influence has come via Christian Western education from the 19th century onwards.

In 1842 the first English speaking Christian missionary arrived at Badagry near Lagos and immediately established a mission, and later the first Western oriented school, near Lagos in 1843.

During the 19th century Western, literary-based education was provided mostly by missionary schools. These schools covered the primary school level and dealt with basic literacy and numeracy. Some secondary schools had also been established. Amongst them were CMS Grammar School Lagos, founded in 1859, and St Gregory's College Lagos, originally a teachers' college, founded in 1878. Other secondary schools and colleges were not directly funded by the missions but by local interested persons. The situation altered considerably in the first part of the 20th century. Emphasis was placed on the acquisition of not only literary but also technical skills. There occurred a large growth of local schools in the coastal areas before the First World War and the establishment of several higher institutes of education like King's College, Lagos, in 1909, Katsina College in 1921, Queen's College, Lagos, in 1927, and the Yaba Higher College in 1934. In parallel with these there existed the traditional Quranic schools in the north of the country.

By the 1930s more emphasis was being placed by Nigerians on secondary schooling. Primary schools were also being built at a high rate in inland areas. The influence of the cities and returning city migrants was quite strong in this respect. A number of students also received education in universities and colleges abroad, in such subjects as engineering, law, sciences, the arts and medicine. Graduates were also trained in medicine at Yaba Higher College.

There occurred a dynamic period of primary school building and a corresponding growth in the school population during the 1950s. In 1955 the Western Region started its free primary education scheme. The Eastern Region followed in 1956. The desire for education amongst Nigerians led to a relatively high degree of literacy amongst ordinary people.

opposite: Art student putting finishing touches to a sculpture at the Yaba College of Technology, Lagos

below: A student sculptor with his work at the Yaba College of Technology in Lagos

Higher education became a key issue of the late 1950s, with the proposal to establish three new universities, namely the University of Nigeria, Nsukka, in the then Eastern Region, and the University of Ife and the Ahmadu Bello University in the then Western and Northern States respectively. Following an invitation in 1959 to Eric Ashby, a former vice-chancellor of Queen's University, Belfast, and his commission's subsequent report, it was decided to set up a system of Higher School Certificates and establish more universities than those three already proposed. The funding of scholarships, especially in technical subjects, by companies such as Shell, also increased, providing more university and college graduates.

In general, the overwhelming desire of Nigerians for education was an important reason why, at Independence, Nigeria was not short of trained technicians in industry and administration. Many other African countries did not find themselves in such a fortunate position.

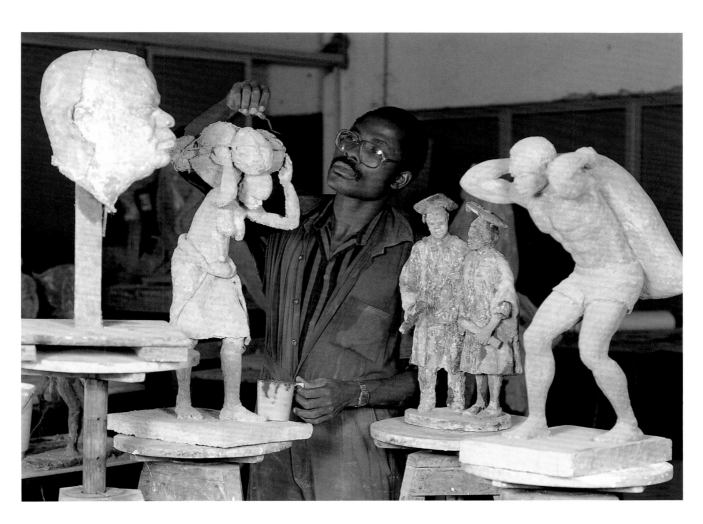

below: The University of Lagos

opposite: In the grounds of an old teacher training college in Katsina

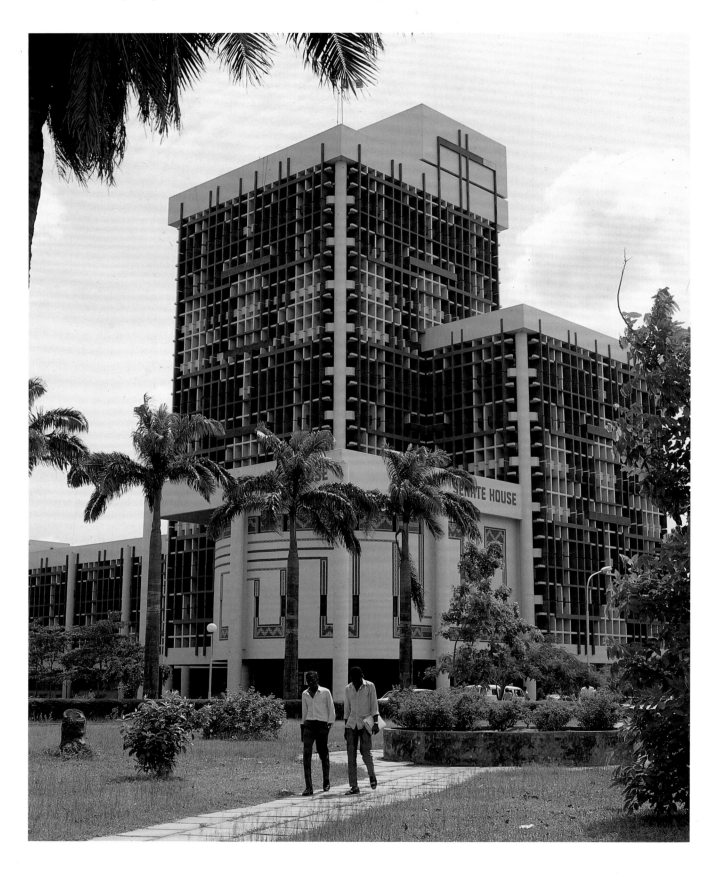

Major, socially responsible companies such as Shell have maintained a broad range of community assistance programmes. Technical and high level manpower required in the oil industry was quite scarce, especially during Shell's pioneering days of oil exploration in Nigeria. Initially the universities were not there to produce the specialists required. Shell therefore offered scholarships to Nigerians to study in universities and colleges of technology overseas. The allocation of more than 1,000 awards has gradually shifted away from overseas universities until the present day when they are given almost exclusively to finance places in Nigerian universities. In addition to research assistance to universities, Shell has also helped to finance construction of buildings and equipment for laboratories. Perhaps the most notable example in this regard was the one million naira granted to Yaba College of Technology in 1960. At the secondary school level, Shell has maintained similar support in the award of scholarships, with the total number exceeding 3,000 at present. In recent years, it has extended its assistance to secondary schools to cover the provision of blocks of classrooms, furniture and laboratory equipment.

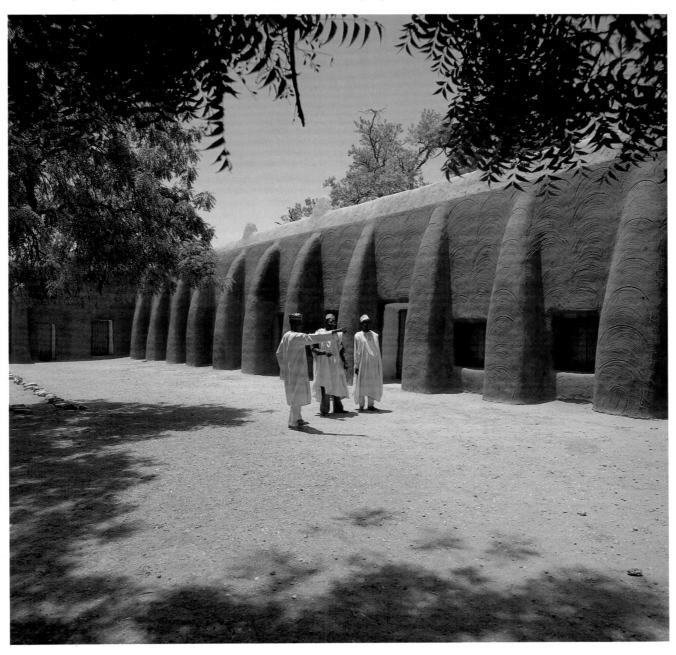

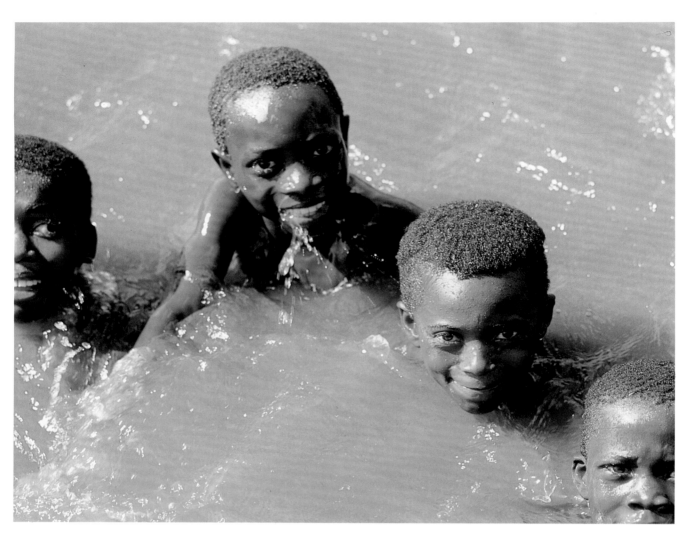

HEALTH

In pre-colonial days, traditional medicine was generally practised throughout the country. Modern medicine was introduced by the British, and this grew with the establishment of clinics and hospitals in various parts of the country, although a large number of Nigerians especially those in the rural areas depended mainly on traditional medicine. The health services in Nigeria have undergone major development and improvement since Nigeria became independent in 1960. Today, modern medicine operates alongside traditional herbal and spiritual medicine in most parts of Nigeria, particularly in the rural areas. The Missionaries Societies have made significant contributions by building hospitals, clinics and providing beds and staff in different parts of the country. In recent times government policy has been to provide modern health services for the total population using primary health care. The main thrust of the Government's plan is to lay emphasis on the control of communicable and endemic diseases through the Expanded Programme on Immunization (EPI), Oral Rehydration Therapy (ORT), basic sanitation and family planning. This health care system is constituted to provide well-defined responsibilities for both the local and state governments for primary and secondary health care respectively. More funding is being provided today by government for the health sector than in the past.

There are 13 Federal Government teaching hospitals providing tertiary care facilities for the training of high level health manpower such as medical doctors, specialist doctors, nurses, medical laboratory technicians and radiographers. In addition, the teaching hospitals provide most of the facilities available in Nigeria today for bio-medical and health research. Four of the teaching hospitals have been designated Centres of Excellence, which indicates that they will provide the best and ultimate facilities for health care, training and research. The University College Hospital Ibadan, the nation's oldest teaching hospital, has been designated the Centre of Excellence in Neurosciences; the University of Nigeria Teaching Hospital for Heart Disease, the University of Maiduguri Teaching Hospital for Infectious Diseases and Ahmadu Bello University Teaching Hospital for Cancer.

opposite: **Children from Ogbe-Ijoh, Bendel State**

below: **The Expanded Programme on Immunisation at the Onikan Health Centre in Lagos**

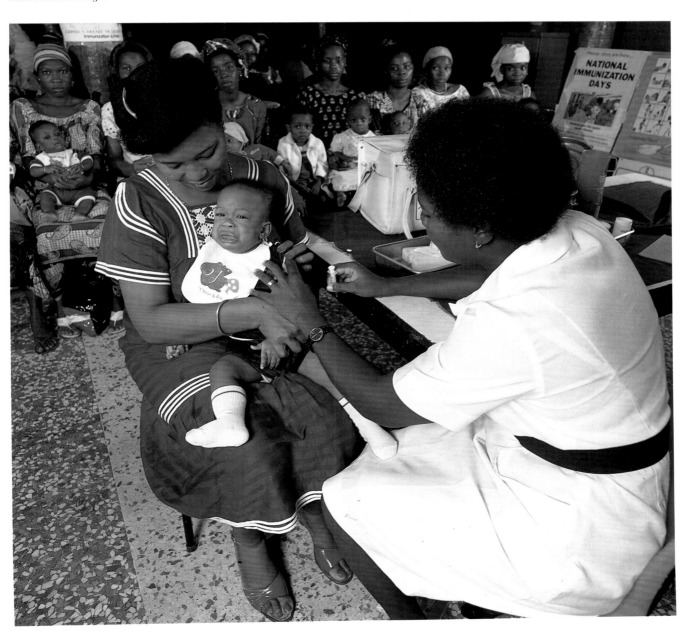